Learning disabilities

Practice issues in health settings

Edited by
Margaret Todd and Tony Gilbert

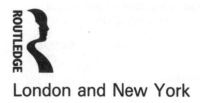

London and New York

First published 1995
by Routledge
11 New Fetter Lane, London EC4P 4EE

Simultaneously published in the USA and Canada
by Routledge
29 West 35th Street, New York, NY 10001

Typeset in English Times by
Pat and Anne Murphy, Highcliffe-on-Sea, Dorset
Printed and bound in Great Britain by
Mackays of Chatham PLC, Chatham, Kent

British Library Cataloguing in Publication Data
A catalogue record for this book is available from
the British Library.

Library of Congress Cataloging in Publication Data
Learning disabilities: practice issues in health setting/edited by
  Margaret Todd and Tony Gilbert.
       p.   cm.
  Includes bibliographical references and index.
  1. Mentally handicapped – Medical care.   2. Mentally
  handicapped – Services for.   3. Learning disabled – Medical care.
  4. Learning disabled – Services for.   I. Todd, Margaret,
  1955–   .   II. Gilbert, Tony, 1956–
  RC570.2.L43   1994   94-1686
  362.2–dc20   CIP

ISBN 0–415–10046–1 (hbk)
ISBN 0–415–10047–X (pbk)

Contents

Illustrations

Contributors

Patricia Brigden B.Sc. (Hons), Dip. Clinical Psychology, Chartered Clinical Psychologist Dip. Management. Consultant Clinical Psychologist, East Berks. (NHS) Trust, for people with a learning disability.

Tony Dix RNMH, ENB 806, Cert. Ed. Nurse Teacher, Southampton University College of Nursing and Midwifery.

Sheila Earwaker RNMH Cert. Ed., Special Education, ENB 806. Nurse Teacher, Basingstoke and Winchester College of Nursing and Midwifery.

Tony Gilbert RNMH, M.Sc., BA, PGCEA. Nurse Teacher, Southampton University College of Nursing and Midwifery, and Professional Nurse Advisor, Learning Disabilities Care Group, Southampton Community Health Service Trust.

Julia Lloyd M.Phil., B.Sc., Dip. Clinical Psychology. Senior Clinical Psychologist. London Community Health Care (NHS) Trust.

Terri Lockyer RNMH, DPNS Cert. Ed. Nurse Teacher, Southampton University College of Nursing and Midwifery.

Margaret Todd RNMH, RMN, RGN, BA (Hons), Dip. Nursing. Nurse Teacher, Buckinghamshire College of Nursing and Midwifery.

Introduction

This book addresses contemporary issues and dilemmas which confront all professionals who work with people with a learning disability. Many of these issues are complex and inter-connected and relate to several different aspects of work in this field.

The book is divided into three parts, which address the issues in relation to social policy and service provision; judgement, decision-making and practice; and finally specific interventions. Each part examines areas which may be considered to be subjects in their own right. However, the concepts contained in the second part crucially underpin or have relevance to the first and last parts. It is therefore recommended that Part II should be read in addition to any other chapter. While many of the concepts contained within this part are particularly complex, their inter-connectedness with the other chapters should be readily apparent. The broad concepts looked at in each part are as follows.

In Part I, the themes of social policy, service provision and levels of intervention raise issues which are considered in relation to the concept of consumerism. This part looks at questions such as who is the consumer, who defines need, and who subsequently determines how these needs will be met. It also looks at how the notion of consumerism relates to the concept of levels of intervention and the development of the professionals employed in providing services for people with a learning disability.

The second part of the book explores the ethical issues related to delivering care and services and the implementation of informed choice and empowerment. Its three chapters are linked by the recurrent theme of paternalism, and the notions of beneficence and non-maleficence. This part considers many of the dilemmas which are encountered by professionals in their day-to-day practice. It does not pretend to offer any easy resolutions to these dilemmas, but provides sufficient insight into the issues to enable practitioners to use this knowledge to inform their practice.

The third and final part of the book focuses on specific behavioural and psychotherapeutic interventions. The issues of paternalism, non-maleficence and empowerment discussed in Part II are of utmost relevance to this part. The main behavioural and psychotherapeutic approaches are explored. While some of the techniques can be considered reductionist, they clearly indicate that the power base lies within the professional domain and are open and honest about this. Other techniques are said to be based on an equal partnership between professional and client, but on closer investigation this may prove not to be the case.

The purpose of this book is to enable the reader to integrate theory into practice. The approach taken in each chapter is first of all to examine the main theoretical concepts and then to explore them further in relation to practice through the presentation of case studies. The case studies are intended to highlight the nature and complexity of the dilemmas practitioners may come up against in day-to-day practice and to help them to consider all the relevant issues in their decision-making. A list of key points is included at the end of each chapter which it is hoped will also be helpful in this respect. Finally, the book ends with a glossary of items additional to those already fully explained in the text.

Part I

Policy and intervention

This first part of the book explores the development of services and professional practice within the context of social policy. The issues raised in the first chapter are illustrated in the development of day services and short-term care services. The historical development of these two services is examined briefly, with a final focus on current service provision. The notion of consumerism is considered within the context of the NHS and Community Care Act 1990 and current service availability.

The concept of consumerism raises the issue of meeting needs. However, before needs can be met they have to be identified and defined so that appropriate services can be developed and provided. A key theme of Chapter 1 is the question, for whom are services developed? Are they developed and provided to meet the needs of individuals with a learning disability, or the needs of their carers/parents or the needs of society? The idea that services may be provided and developed to meet the needs of professional staff is also addressed. At first sight, this last idea may seem surprising. However, in looking at how needs are defined, it becomes apparent that it is professional staff who play the key role in identifying and subsequently meeting needs they themselves have defined. It remains to be seen what impact the NHS and Community Care Act 1990 will have on this situation.

In addition to the development of service provision, Chapter 2 explores the development of professional involvement in the lives of people with a learning disability. Since the two main statutory service providers are the Health Service and the local authority through social services departments, the roles of the nurse for people with a learning disability and the social worker are examined in depth. This examination is set in the context of the welfare state and the concept of the 'deserving and undeserving poor'. The purpose of Part I is to unpack the complexity of health and social care provision for learning disabled people in the the context of community care and care management. Its two chapters form the base for the remainder of the book as they place the provision of contemporary services and issues firmly within a historical and social policy perspective.

Chapter 1

Services for people with a learning disability

Sheila Earwaker and Margaret Todd

INTRODUCTION

Services for people with learning disabilities have grown and developed during the twentieth century. Journals are full of examples of 'good practice'. Professionals and their organisations take pride in highlighting their centres of excellence for the benefit of those service providers who have not made the same progress with their own service developments. Centres of excellence offer their ideas so that less developed services can pick up useful tips. Traditionally, services were designed by professionals who decided what the client needed; these have developed into businesses which continually strive to seek new growth and to support professionals in need of an income. As stated by McKnight (1981), the business of modern society is service, and social service in modern society is business. Services now boast of more, and better educated, staff. There is a wide variety of service provision and experience available to assist people with learning disabilities. Professionals in the area include teachers, residential and community nurses, social workers and psychologists.

Services have developed more in-depth methods of assessing needs, have become more adept at defining those needs and employ professionals who are becoming increasingly skilled in producing solutions to assessed and defined needs. They are currently re-organising in an attempt to provide better systems for delivering the solutions to those needs. There is now an expanding, competitive market where superior cost-effective services are being sought for people. Legislation has recently been enacted which supports this economy (Department of Health 1990). These are encouraging signs, and surely a recipe for well-matched, appropriate services to be delivered in a professional and rational way.

However, one outcome of this growing and developing business of service is that there are ever-increasing demands to be met, an ever-increasing budget to be found to pay for the service, and a continuing reluctance on the part of society to support the cost of providing such services. For the individuals who use the services, there appears to be some dissonance between the amount of energy, research and funding put into their delivery, and the quality of the goods received in return. The last two decades have introduced and promoted the principles of normalisation and community care alongside the philosophy of the open market, three major factors in the evolution of services to people with learning disabilities. These developments are all aimed at improving the service offered, but how well are the service providers putting the theory into practice?

The nature of the service provision is determined by both professional and political considerations. Professionals continue to define need but in a much more competitive arena, and by defining need influence those responsible for determining service delivery. At the same time there are limitations on resources, and it is not possible to meet all identified needs. The resulting situation is one in which services do not always provide what people want, or need, because the design, organisation and delivery of the services is not simply a matter for negotiation between recipient and provider (Macdonald 1991). Factors which affect the situation include: who defines the needs of the service users and the solutions to those needs; how much money will be available for the services; the limitations imposed by the current service providers in terms of their conventional ideas about what should be available; and the amount of finance tied up in current provision.

Recent governments have produced policy documents regarding services to people with learning disabilities making recommendations for their development, and these documents have offered some consistency over the years. The consistency has been in their failure to specify exact goals, while maintaining a commitment to improve quality and decrease costs (Baldwin 1991). The effect of not specifying goals is that there is no measure of failure. Moreover, a commitment to improve quality would result in increased cost, at least temporarily. This would suggest a lack of real intent to improve the situation.

This chapter shows how the current state of provision has been arrived at by following the development of two specific services. While there are many service examples which could be used for illustration, the provision of day services and short-term care services to people with learning disabilities highlights the issues involved particularly clearly.

CONSUMERISM

One of the key issues in the NHS reforms is that of consumer choice (Mooney 1992). It is assumed that the best judges of consumer preference are the consumers themselves. It is stated that consumer choice should determine which services will be provided (Mooney *et al.* 1986). In fact the consumers of the health service are probably the least powerful group able to influence health care. The National Health Service has never been sensitive to the services users' views and desires (Royal College of Nursing 1988). The power to determine service provision is most strongly influenced by the professionals and service providers who define need and provide services to meet these needs.

The philosophy of consumerism assumes that the service user is well-informed about the range and type of service available. It also assumes that consumers are able and willing to make decisions regarding the service they want (Mooney 1992), and that a diversity of provision exists. The political commitment to the market economy underlying the concept of consumerism leads to the belief that people will purchase only those services that they want or need and that market forces will thus determine the provision of services.

These assumptions are not necessarily true in relation to health care, where people can only purchase the service that is available, even if it does not fully satisfy their needs. In fact, the consumer model reinforces the argument that what is already provided is what people want, because they continue to purchase it. Consumers are not always well-informed about the services that are available, and there are still not many competing suppliers of services, particularly for learning disabled people. The further assumption that service users have the necessary knowledge and skills to articulate their demands (Mooney *et al.* 1986) may not be the case for people with a learning disability, who may need an advocate to assist them. It is claimed that the final decision regarding which services should be provided in health care will inevitably remain in the hands of professionals and government, because consumers do not know what services they want or need (Mooney *et al.* (1986).

This is a surprising statement. In the field of learning disabilities some consumers of services have been voicing their wants and needs quite clearly over a number of years, although so far services have failed to respond adequately. This issue will be explored in relation to day services and short-term care services.

DAY SERVICES

The concept of day services for adults with learning disabilities in Britain is a relatively recent development in health and social services provision. The earliest responsibilities for such provision were placed on local councils and boroughs under the 1890 Lunacy Act, which charged them with providing institutional and community services to people with learning disabilities. Community services were limited to what was provided under the Poor Law of 1601, supplemented by the work of voluntary bodies (NDG 1977b). The 1913 Mental Deficiency Act specifically tackled the provision of training, occupation and supervision, but the intervention of the First World War delayed progress in this area and 'occupation centres' for people classified as mentally defective slowly emerged between the First and Second World Wars.

Until 1948, local authorities had a duty to provide 'supervision' and training for occupation for those not living in institutions, and institutions for those who could not be cared for at home (DHSS 1971). The National Health Service Act (1946) allowed for the provision of training centres by local authorities, although during the 1950s and 1960s most junior and adult training centres were the responsibility of health authorities. However, it was not until the report of the Royal Commission on the Law Relating to mental Illness and Mental Deficiency (1957), which promoted care in the community, that it was felt necessary to include a duty to provide training centres as a feature of the Mental Health Act of 1959. This was later reinforced by the National Health Service Act of 1977.

Little can be established about the purpose of these centres, although it is assumed that they are intended solely to provide a supervised form of occupation, which was in some way productive. Traditional adult training centre (ATC) 'trainees' were engaged in assembly work, but there was a growing movement during the 1960s which favoured the educationalist views of Tizard, Gunzberg and Clarke (Hancock 1988). The first investment in the staff working in these centres was made when a teacher training programme was developed in 1964. The Ministry of Health produced a *Good Practice Guide* in 1968, which suggested that training was about developing specific work habits and continuing schooling, and this view supported the notion that 'teachers' were the appropriate staff to have in such centres.

During this time, foundations were being laid to promote a service for people with learning disabilities that centred on 'schooling' and training for work. It may be a reflection of the success that people were achieving in the area of their 'schooling' that prompted a major swing away from the view that such people were ineducable. The magnitude of the swing became evident in the 1970 Education Act, which gave responsibility to the local education authorities for the education of all children, including those with severe handicaps. The junior training centres became special schools overnight, often without a change of premises or staff for several years. While the immediate changes in responsibility and labelling may have indicated the government's commitment to progress, the finance required to provide educational material and suitably qualified staff was much later in arriving.

This resulted in a slightly different function for the adult training centres as described by the DHSS in its 1971 report. Leaving out the notion of 'schooling', but indicating the provision of further training and daily occupation, it describes centres as aiming to develop work habits and increase self-reliance. The inclusion of the provision of occupation as an aim is important, as this may have been an honest evaluation of what the centres were actually providing for people. Since almost all trainees in most adult training centres could expect to stay for the rest of their lives (Carter 1981), the question of the value of training to the trainee is one which has frequently been raised, and rarely satisfactorily answered. Perhaps another factor in the confusion over the role which these services were undertaking may have been the different meanings attached to the terms 'education' and 'training'. In addition, the staff working in the services may have been given the brief to train people for work, but not the brief to move people on from where they were. The result of well-meant but unclear intentions was to produce a situation in which people viewed attendance at centres as:

(a) a long-term career move for the learning disabled person;
(b) a *fait accompli* for the social worker who found the place;

(c) a move which would eventually lead to a silting-up of placements.

It is therefore not surprising to find that the DHSS report (1971)
recommended that provision should be increased from 25,000
places in 1970 to 74,000 places in the 1990s.

The move towards community care

During the 1970s, local authorities seemed to develop an almost
exclusive provision of day services which had often been initiated
by voluntary agencies, or transferred during the frequent reorgan-
isations of health and social services taking place at that time.
Under the NHS Act of 1977 they became obliged to provide such
services within the resources available. Training centres were seen
as a positive move from institutional to community care. This is
surprising, since many day services were sited in the grounds of
institutions, or in 'residential areas' (where the residents might well
be elsewhere during the operational hours of the service). This
would have offered little opportunity for contact with the community. The increase in size of such centres, from an average of
eighty-five places in the 1960s to 120 places in 1973 (Carter 1981),
also suggests that centres were not so much pursuing the notion of
community care as maintaining the elements of institutional care.

Teasdale (1989) proposes that the idea of community care, and
day services themselves, arose from the change in attitude to institutions fuelled by evidence which presented them in a very negative
light. However, the development of day services which 'meet' the
needs of people by providing services within a unit where clients
attend and staff work, perpetuates the values of institutional care.
Although day centres are not 'total institutions' as defined by
Goffman (1961), at this time they showed several of the features he
ascribes to such institutions, the most important being the social
distance that was created between staff and clients. This may still
be the case in some services today, but it is usually more subtle in
nature. A guiding principle of supervision rather than sharing is
usually indicative of the maintenance of power over 'trainees' and
is recognised as such by people with learning disabilities, who
resent the authority of staff (Jahoda et al. 1989).

The National Development Group (1977b) reinforced the belief
that such centres were to be the key resource in the community, and

placed the emphasis of need back on education. This was a change from the original function of assembly work, and was in keeping with the recent developments in staff training in the field of teaching, and a slight change from the DHSS (1971) view of their purpose as one of occupation and training.

A survey carried out during 1974–8 found that the staff wanted more education classes, arts and crafts, increased social activities, discussion groups and so on (Carter 1981), and these findings confirmed a combined approach to the educational direction for training centres, which were to become known as social education centres (SECs). The same survey also identified that users of the services wanted more work activities, but although this finding was included in the NDG (1977b) report, it was not considered paramount. The title of 'student' ascribed to users reflected the educational emphasis of the new service approach, despite a clear statement in the report that the client group included people whose need for day services is as much a function of the local employment and economic situation as of any inherent learning disability. This conflicted with other views held at the time, which suggested that users of day services were outside the open labour market or were economically inactive (Carter 1981).

The function of day services

The task of staff was described in the report as one of facilitating educational development in the individual and group, and was concerned with every aspect of personal competence and development. Functions of the service were described as:

(a) admission and assessment;
(b) development and activities;
(c) special care;
(d) advanced work.

There was an intention that, for people who could progress from (a) to (d), there would be an opportunity to move on to employment schemes and/or jobs (a throughput model). Individuals could be referred to centres by a variety of people, including the education authority, family, social worker, consultant or disablement resettlement officer. The NDG (1977b) recommended that every entrant was to be assessed, so that needs could be identified and matched to what the centre had to offer. This is striking in that it reflects the idea that any person with learning disabilities will be a suitable client for the service, and also that an individual's needs will be able to 'fit in' to what is being offered. It would seem that people were not assessed to see what a service should provide, but to see where they could be slotted into an existing service.

In practice, there did appear to be entry criteria for a day placement. Many people who had agressive or disruptive behaviour, incontinence or an inability to walk had been denied places in day centres. Day activities for people with severe learning disabilities and additional special needs, who were living in the community, were to be provided for within special care units attached to such centres. When facilities were made available to this group of people, they were not always as well provided for as the NDG (1977b) had envisaged. Allen (1990) describes a study conducted by Norris of eighty-one people in five special care units which produced largely negative findings: inadequate physical facilities, poor standard of equipment, low and insufficient staffing and poor back-up support. Perhaps one of the more significant beliefs of the NDG (1977b) was that most recommendations could be implemented at relatively low cost. This was in line with the assumption made in the Education Act (1970) and the National Health Service Act (1988) that recommended changes could and should take place without extra finance.

Following publication of the NDG Report (1977b), many centres expanded their services to encompass a diversity and variety of provision. At the same time social services departments were under pressure to extend their services whilst being under-funded and under-staffed. During the 1980s, SECs again changed their title, this time to day service, and training for staff began to take place through social work qualifications, such as the Certificate in Social Services or the Certificate in Qualified Social Work and, more recently, the Diploma in Social Work. This suggests that the services were now responding to a need identified as one with a social as well as an educational dimension and to some extent explains the preoccupation with the use of community facilities such as sports centres, local shops and hostelries to carry out the functions of the service. These activities may offer evidence that the service is carrying out its functions in keeping with the philosophy and principles of normalisation. However, the fact that normalisation might imply rejection of the idea of offering such a service at all, and for so large a number of people, makes this a very difficult idea to understand. A MENCAP publication (1985) identifies this as one of the major problems attached to basing a service on such principles, and the same problem is also apparent in the various definitions of normalisation and its goals. Wolfensberger (1972) offers the definition of using means which are culturally normative as far as possible to establish and/or maintain behaviours which are as culturally normative as possible.

While services enthusiastically professed themselves to be under the influence of normalisation, they often did so without pausing to consider the meaning behind the philosophy. MENCAP (1985) suggests that the phrase 'as far as possible' provides one of the major difficulties in transferring the ideology into practice, but that it is a challenge which cannot be rejected. Another difficulty in applying the philsophy of normalisation is that in practice it limits the person to passively receiving services. Neither is it clear whether patterns of everyday living are means to an end or an end state in themselves (Hattersley 1991). Yet another view is that normalisation results in the imposition of a particular way of life on a particular group of people. Despite the disagreement about the meaning of normalisation, the clients and staff of services are to be congratulated on the achievements they have made in the much debated area of social integration. ATCs and SECs have gone a long way towards widening the activities and initiatives for people with learning disabilities.

It is difficult to apply the principles of normalisation, or social role valorisation, if day services are to be 'all things to all men'. Jahoda et al. (1989) reported that although services have introduced and adapted various initiatives, there is still a debate about whether services should have an educational focus or be based on work experience with the aim of employment. Having a job is one of the basic activities that most people strive for in our society today, but day services offer little tie-up with careers services or re-assessment for other schemes (Nelson 1989). They currently appear to have an almost impossible task, which is to provide each individual with a range of programmes for assessed need in the areas of leisure, recreation, social education, domestic skills and employment. Seed (1988) describes seven different models of day service provision, with associated aims, based on research conducted in 1984:

1 The work model: to provide work experience and, where possible, preparation for employment.

2 The social care model: to provide social education, such as to develop normal living potential and social skills needed in a family and community context.
3 The further education model: to provide continuing education to develop adult potential.
4 The throughput model: to channel people to more appropriate (more normal) placements including preparation for employment.
5 The recreation model: to provide opportunities to develop individual potential through a range of interests and activities.
6 The shared living model: to provide opportunities for shared learning.
7 The resource centre model: to meet a variety of client and community needs, as a resource centre.

While some services concentrate on one particular function, many services are attempting to provide most or all of these programmes with a staff–client ratio of 1:15. The result of combining several different and usually separate functions in one service in one place is that it stretches the skill and energy of the staff to the point where little is achieved or done well (Harper 1989). It may seem more appropriate to offer a range of services based in different environments, depending on the activities pursued, funded by the appropriate bodies such as education, employment and social services.

Restructuring

Schemes are developing across the country in an attempt to resolve this issue. An early example was Blake's Wharf in Hammersmith, West London, an employment agency which emerged as a separate service from the ATC but was funded by the local social services department. Similar agencies are becoming more available, and organisations such as the Shaw Trust assist financially in the promotion of paid work for people with learning disabilities. However, there is little acknowledgement of such agencies as work-training schemes because they come under the remit of social services rather than employment services. The view is maintained that they are a substitute service for the real thing. At the same time they have the real effect of keeping unemployment figures down.

Seed (1988) proposes that the strengths of day care could be combined in three new models of provision – Work, Further Education and Community Resource – replacing the original seven. However, even though employment and education agencies are involved in the provision of the services described, each of the three models still relies heavily on the social services departments as the key agency.

The recommendations of the Social Services Inspectorate (SSI) (1989) and the government guidelines (Department of Health 1990) for the development of day services for people with learning disabilities, offer little in the way of change. They imply that social services departments will still be responsible for the assessment and regular re-assessment of client needs, maintaining the potential for re-interpretation of needs if they do not fit the services currently on offer. Provision is to be developed following the principles of community care (as resources allow), despite recognition in the SSI report that, although staff talk of community care, normalisation and highest potential, few appear to understand the implications of these ideas for their role and tasks.

Many local authorities are again restructuring their day services in an attempt to provide more integrated activities for the people they serve, and to act as more of a resource centre. There is a definite move away from the idea of separate buildings for ATCs and a strengthening of the 'integrating' activities available to the rest of the population. Some day services continue to employ teaching staff, as well as a wide range of other staff with qualifications in a trade or other relevant backgrounds such as psychology.

Restructuring has been a constant feature in some centres, and outreach work, involvement in further education establishments and satellite units are becoming more commonplace (Durrant 1989). Centres are now facing closure, with services offering base units only and clients using generic facilities. However, until the question of purpose is resolved, the energy and finances involved in constant change may well prove unproductive. If restructuring is to be effective, then there needs to be a clear sense of purpose and concentration on one area of activity. The King's Fund reported (1980) that the first priority for constructing a good quality day service is to establish its purpose. This is apparently contradicted, in a later publication (King's Fund 1984), which in discussing the fact that day services are over-stretched, begins by talking about the need for a model rather than a purpose. It states that a decision must be taken as to whether a traditional model of day provision is wanted or something more in line with emerging thinking on community participation. One might question what purpose either model would serve, and also whose purposes might influence the decision. However, the paper then moves on to develop a clear case for a vocational service, based on the goals of equal rights and participation, informed and supported by the views of people with learning disabilities.

The question of which and whose needs are being served by day services also needs to be addressed. Schneider (1990) identified the following groups and needs:

• Health and welfare personnel: for monitoring/follow-up, containment, control, protection, advice, counselling, rehabilitation and medication.
• Residental care staff: for diversion.
• Relatives: for respite.
• Society: for containment.
• Users: for the satisfaction of physiological and psychological needs.

Perhaps, then, the most important thing to be clear about is the purpose of provision. If it is true that day services are to serve the needs of a whole host of other people in addition to the people with learning disabilities, then providers need to be explicit about their aims, and abandon the claim that such services are in keeping with the principles of normalisation. If, on the other hand, the purpose is to provide for the people with learning disabilities, then the voice of these people should be listened to, heard and then responded to with equal emphasis. Unfortunately, the emphasis tends to be very much on listening: many authors report that people who currently attend day services express the wish for a real job, but their voice still seems relatively unheard. Jahoda et al. (1989) established that the people most concerned were grateful to have somewhere to go, enjoyed the sociable atmosphere and the learning of skills, but also identified that they were aware of the substitution for real work, resented the authority of staff, and were hurt by the stigma associated with attending an ATC. Table 1.1 provides a summary of the policies that have affected day service provision to date.

The future

Are we able to admit, after so much hard work by so many people, at a very great cost, that what is still provided for the majority of people with a learning disability is occupation, and what is provided

Table 1.1 Policy influencing day service provision

Instrument	Policy
1890 Lunacy Act	Local councils and boroughs to provide institutional and community services.
1913 Mental Deficiency Act	Provision of training, occupation and supervision.
1946 NHS Act	Local authorities could fund training centres.
1959 Mental Health Act	Local authorities must provide training centres.
1968 Good Practice Guide	To provide training for specific work habits/schooling.
1970 Education Act	Children to attend school (now seen as educable!).
1971 White Paper	Centres to develop work habits and self-reliance.
1977 NDG Report No. 5	Centres for education: assessment, development, activities, advanced work.
1989 Social Services Inspectorate	Centres for assessment and re-assessment. Social services departments retain responsibility.

for their carers is respite? To be effective, change has to be directed at the entire system (Blunden 1991). A system has been developed for provision of day services that undergoes regular change, but after many years of modifications, there appears to be little fundamental difference to the overall provision. While the stated aims for services might – if they were achievable – be admirable, there must be some concern for the clients and staff of such services, since these aims are not reflected in the outcomes for people. This must be increasingly frustrating for all individuals concerned. The government have been happy to finance the collection of information and the writing of several reports, which indicate the path to follow in the provision of day services for people with a learning disability. While these guidelines are not coherent with what the services are attempting to do, they consistently offer approval of what people are actually doing now. This avoids the necessity for providing any significantly different or more expensive options.

Reports are published recommending a particular direction for services only after that direction has been followed by service leaders. The NDG (1977b) recommended that training centres should become education centres more than ten years after staff began training as teachers; the White Paper *Caring for People* (Great Britain 1989) recommended that institutional settings be replaced in favour of community settings, again some years after day services had begun attempting to do this. The government guidelines (Department of Health 1990) recommend a service provision based on individual assessments and programme plans, supporting individual development, something most services have already been doing for several years.

One interpretation of this very uninspiring guidance might be that the intention is to deliberately slow down any significant change. Services are having to struggle to take the next step. Policy-makers wait until this has almost been achieved before reviewing progress and direction and then, if they approve, authorise a report recommending that the way forward should be exactly what the services are already doing.

It seems that overall the future for day services will be very similar to the present situation, which in turn bears a very strong resemblance to provision in the past. It is evident that, for a small number of people in successful areas, things are very different. For example, consortia have been set up in some places adopting a service-brokerage approach whereby individuals receiving care are given money to purchase the services they wish. The impact of advocacy schemes has resulted in people demanding from providers the services they require, and in many cases this has been work. However, for the majority of people attending day services, there has been little real change. The *raison d'être* may well seem different, in that we change from claiming to provide occupation, to providing education, training and preparation for living in the community and for employment, to whatever the next politically correct assumption is. The environment may also change from large centres to more potentially integrative small units, but this in itself is not the answer to the dilemma of purpose. The staff may undergo a different form of training, but unless radical change occurs, day services for people with a learning disability will remain essentially the same.

SHORT-TERM CARE SERVICES

'Respite care' is an expression, frequently used these days, often intended to carry the same meaning as the terms 'short-term care', 'phased care', 'relief care', 'planned care', 'programmed care', 'holiday care', 'social admission' and 'shared care'. Respite care, however, has a particular meaning which some of the other terms do not reflect: 'respite – a delay in the discharge of an obligation or suffering of a penalty; interval of rest or relief' (*Oxford English Dictionary* 1964).

This term has recently become very fashionable, largely replacing 'short-term care' which was the term used from the 1960s to the 1980s. Oswin (1984) defined short-term care as being arrangements whereby people with a learning disability are looked after in a place other than their home for a short period of time not exceeding two or three months. This definition merely states the arrangements in care, as opposed to implying reasons for care. Since the word 'respite' has overtones of burden, it might seem more appropriate to re-institute the term 'short-term care'.

The development of short-term care as a service

Government policies have to some extent influenced the provision of short-term care services over the last forty years, but the leap from recognition of need to adequate provision has not yet been achieved. According to Oswin (1984), the concept of short-term care was first recognised officially in 1952 by the DHSS in a circular which recommended the use of this form of care, paid for in part or in full by local health authorities.

At that time, this care had been provided unofficially for children in the wards of hospitals for people with a learning disability, in order to give families relief. Following this official recognition of need, there was a steady increase in the numbers of people admitted for short-term care to hospitals for people with a learning disability, and this process was itself followed by a procedure of 'informal admission' permitted by the Mental Health Act 1959 (DHSS 1959). During the 1960s and 1970s, this arrangement continued, with the NHS providing the majority of places for children in paediatric wards of general hospitals, and for both children and adults in hospitals for people with a learning disability. There were some disturbing reports of poor standards of care for long-stay residents in hospitals about this time, but despite this the number of short-term care admissions doubled during the 1970s. The options for carers remained limited, as neither local authority, nor voluntary, nor private resources were plentiful or easily accessible.

The Education Act of 1970 was a significant piece of legislation which may have directly affected the call for short-term care. Prior to this act, children with severe learning disabilities were deemed uneducable and were not considered suitable for schooling, but were sometimes offered places at junior training centres where places were available. Parents of those who could not secure a place were often advised to put their children into full-time residential care. Following the act, more parents may have been able to care for their child at home, since education was made available to all children regardless of the severity of their handicap. The daily provision for all children may have been the help needed to encourage parents to continue the full-time care themselves. In addition, there was the hope and expectation provided by recognition of the child's ability to develop – a major stimulus for the carers. Other influences may have included the timely provision of attendance allowances and mobility allowances, made available through the Chronically Sick and Disabled Persons Act 1970. This gave recognition to the fact that people with disabilities required constant attention and help with mobility, but although financially helpful to carers, the benefits did not reflect the enormous amount of time and energy that some parents and families were expending, without other practical support.

In 1971 the government produced a document (DHSS 1971) on what special help was required for the individuals concerned, what was being done for them at the time, and what ought to be done in the future. The report recognised that families required help which was rarely available, and referred to the limited provision by local authorities of short-term care for both children and adults. The recommendations included provision of short-term care places in existing homes for people with learning disabilities, the use of foster parents and guesthouse proprietors, and possibly seasonal provision for holidays. Having acknowledged that caring for relatives at home makes great calls on emotional reserves, the extent of reference in the report to short-term care seems relatively insignificant.

The influence of community workers

The creation of social service departments in 1971 may also have been seen as a development in the provision of services, since the Seebohm Report of 1968 recommended that these departments should be responsible for a comprehensive range of services for people with learning disabilities in the community. The social worker, according to the 1971 White Paper (DHSS 1971), was the person best placed to co-ordinate the services of a multi-disciplinary team, providing services which would include counselling and practical assistance. However, by the late 1970s, a growing number of community nurses for people with a learning disability appeared in these multi-disciplinary teams, who provided advice and emotional support to carers and may also have had some influence on the uptake of short-term care. One of the roles of both the community nurse and the social worker is to prevent the need for long-term care by providing carers with enough support for them to manage at home. The promotion of short-term care to parents may have been a result of the emerging philosophy of community care and the belief that people should live in their own homes with adequate support. Alternatively, it could have been due to the fact that most hospitals for people with learning disabilities were full and could not reasonably grow any more. Long-term care was becoming increasingly difficult to acquire, and short-term care could provide a temporary solution to some families' difficulties.

While the outcome for the carers and clients may not prove significantly different, the reason behind the provision of the service is entirely different. In the first instance, the service is offered in the belief that this is the best provision for the individual and/or family, whereas in the second, the service is offered as an alternative because the original service is no longer available. Of course, the development of short-term care as an acceptable option may have occurred as a result of both influences. While it may seem difficult to separate these influences, it is interesting to note that the notion of community care had been around for some years (it was developed by the Royal Commission in 1957), but that alternative services became available only when existing services became unable to cope with demand.

Some community nurses and social workers may well have been in the position of 'selling' short-term care to families (despite the families' reluctance), the service being something concrete that they could offer. Oswin (1984) describes some parents' initial reactions to the use of short-term care in negative terms. These responses might imply that short-term care was not something that was initiated by all carers, but offered as a solution to other difficulties encountered. Sloper and Turner (1992) suggest that respite care services have become a useful answer to stressful demands which services have been unable to respond to by alleviating them in another way. Short-term care will not relieve problems created by poor housing, low wages and unemployment, and the individual with learning disabilities in a family may be scapegoated as the source of the problem, so avoiding deeper social issues (Oswin 1984).

Short-term care for the carers

Short-term care is a service which creates a certain amount of stress in itself. It can be difficult to book a place when required, impossible to access at short notice, be some distance away, difficult to organise transport, or not suitable for the person being cared for. Short-term care is frequently offered with all the emphasis on the benefits for the carers, that is, how wonderful it would be for the carers to have some time to themselves, have a break, go out and socialise. Even though carers may have mentioned some negative effects of short-term care on themselves and for the individual concerned, this tends to have been ignored.

Short-term care is chiefly promoted as giving parents a break from looking after a difficult or tiring child or dependent adult, and is based on the idea of burden. This interpretation is a common one, usually used by professionals when defining the problem. While some parents would agree, many feel anxious about leaving their child or dependent adult with others, and are not solely concerned with their own escape from caring. Hubert (1991) describes the experiences and perceptions of twenty different families whose concerns are about the physical, emotional and intellectual well-being and happiness of their children or dependent adults. The decision to accept offers of short-term care is not made easily, many parents reporting feelings of guilt and inadequacy. There may also be a lack of confidence in other people's ability to interpret the individual's needs and wants. Pressure used to persuade parents may devalue their efforts to cope alone, as so many had to do for years without appropriate support.

Anderson (1982), however, believes that initial resistance from parents is due to the fear that short-term care may be the start of the slippery slope leading to rejection, and offers the view that total responsibility may be easier for parents than partial responsibility. He also suggests that parents fear that other carers will do better than they, and are anxious that any peculiar ways they have of dealing with the child may become public knowledge. Anderson (1982) does not go on to consider that some care staff may appreciate knowledge of alternative ways of managing care, and that the parents' years of dealing with particular (or peculiar) situations may have produced creative solutions.

Although Oswin (1984) reported that parents had no help in coping with the emotional upheaval in using short-term care services, community teams for people with learning disabilities not only promote its provision, but also claim to support the families during this difficult time. Perhaps in 1984 there were not as many community teams in existence, maybe the support offered cannot reduce the emotional impact, or possibly the professionals are not the right people to be offering the support required. In addition to professional help and advice, there are various other systems available to individual carers which are just as, if not more, important than the professional opinion. These include the family's neighbours, local community and work/recreation associates. The views of this group may influence greatly either the decision to use short-term care or the emotional reaction to the decision made.

Short-term care does have its benefits for carers. It has been suggested that it offers carers the opportunity to recharge their batteries, spend time with their other children or spouse, have a holiday, be selfish, attend to other taks, relieve stress, prevent breakdown, sleep, or cover emergencies such as accident or illness.

Short-term care for the individual

If these are the experiences of the parents and carers when their relative takes up the provision, what are the experiences for the person with the learning disability? Short-term care during the 1970s was largely based on the carer's viewpoint and on the basis of relief. The function in relation to assessment and rehabilitation was a secondary consideration. As well as being promoted to the carer as relief, it was also sometimes 'sold' to the individual as a holiday. This may have been a valid point, since some people may well have been keen to experience a new or different environment, with a range of different people. For the individual receiving the service, short-term care potentially offers:

(a) a change of surroundings;
(b) the opportunity for assessment;
(c) attention to health problems;
(d) active rehabilitation of many kinds;
(e) the opportunity to take a break from being with parents;
(f) the opportunity to continue to live at home;
(g) the opportunity to increase their social networks;
(h) the opportunity for personal growth and enjoyment.

These are the likely factors which may be put to the individual with learning disabilities when short-term care is suggested as an option, and indeed some schemes did cater for some of these needs. However, a study carried out in 1984 by Ayer and Alaszewski suggested that there was little evidence of short-term care being used for more than the relief of parents. If this is the case, then further consideration must be given to the experiences of the person with the learning disability.

There can be a variety of negative effects for the person receiving care: separation can be traumatic for both parties. It may be difficult to explain what is happening, and the individual may well be unsettled. This may be demonstrated by a change in the individual's usual behaviours, and frustration or disturbed behaviour may be attributed to the nature of the disability instead of changing circumstances (Anderson 1982). A mourning response may be elicited, and home-sickness may be experienced, in addition to feeling a sense of rejection and insecurity.

One answer to the difficulties raised here is provided by a gradual introduction to the environment and staff group. This has the benefit of building up relationships, by slowly increasing the time spent in the new environment. One of the dilemmas which remains unresolved, however, is where the needs of the individual and the carer conflict. Carers may be in need of some assistance with the care of the individual; they may be unwell or have other commitments which demand time and attention; the individual, however, may not want to leave his or her own home because of this.

The provision

The National Development Group (1977a), while agreeing that short-term care was not easy to define, suggested that it referred to the admission of persons with a learning disability to a residential unit on the understanding that they would return to their previous address within a short period of time. The use of residential units for this form of care was confirmed by the view that short-term care should be seen not only as a temporary relief from the burdens of care (although this is valuable), but that it should also be used to service the need for assessment and treatment. The emphasis of this document, while recognising that fostering or 'boarding out' does occur in some authorities, is on providing short-term care in existing residential units, thus maintaining the significance of professional intervention. The report states that planning should begin with an appraisal of resources already available within the NHS local authority and voluntary agencies, and refers to current expenditure restraint. This course of action, aimed at keeping things the way they were, may have reflected the lack of priority given to any improvements in the provision of short-term care.

The following year, however, the Warnock Report (Department of Education and Science 1978) recommended that a variety of forms of short-term relief should be available to parents of children with severe disabilities who live at home, and this was the first indication that real changes were intended to occur. One option proposed was that there should be opportunity for someone other than the parent to look after the child at home for part of the day, or for one or two days, under a befriending scheme. Another option recommended was short-term fostering where the person with the learning disability is cared for in the home of another family. The Jay report (DHSS 1979) confirmed the view that a variety of options should be available, and described the provision needed as that offering domiciliary care of a wide-ranging kind from a short time to several weeks. Rapid growth in short-term care facilities occurred during the late 1970s, organised by local authorities, health authorities and voluntary and parents' groups. The fostering scheme mentioned in the Warnock Report (Department of Education and Science 1978) was developed, since it could be funded under the provisions of the Health and Public Services Act (1968), which enabled local authorities to meet the costs. However, much of the provision was still being provided away from the family home, and depended on the person with the learning disability moving out for the period of time negotiated by the carer. The services were mainly being offered:

(a) by the NHS in learning disabilities hospitals;
(b) by the NHS in paediatric wards;
(c) by the NHS in assessment centres;
(d) by the NHS in residential homes;
(e) by the local authority in children's and adults' hostels;
(f) by the education authority in hostels attached to special schools;
(g) by voluntary agencies in their homes.

Some purpose-built units were emerging, while other services offered a few places within the existing residential care provision. For the individuals who are involved in these forms of provision, there is a world of difference. It is one thing to attend a residential facility where there is a group of people all there for similar reasons. It is quite another to live in someone else's home for a few days, and be an enforced visitor.

Some schemes appeared, such as Crossroads and voluntary groups, which offered assistance within the individual's home, but these were scarce and often difficult to access. During the 1980s, there was an increase in family placements for people with learning disabilities. Various names were given to such schemes – 'fostering', 'family link', 'adult placement' and so on. These placements, however, which were available to both children and adults, were often restricted to people who had the least disadvantages. Hubert (1991) found that residential units were often the only form of service available for individuals with severe or multiple disabilities.

Stalker (1991) reported that black and ethnic minority families were more likely to receive short-term care through institutional provision, and Duff (1992) referred to three families who were excluded from short-term care services because of challenging behaviour, and the need for one-to-one staffing.

Caring for People (Great Britain 1989) set out the intention to develop a wide range of services to be provided in a variety of settings, and described the availability of short-term care to assist carers as essential. There was no reference to extra funds being made available to assist this development, and again, the emphasis in the definition of respite care was put upon alternative accommodation. There have been several reports on preference for care which indicate that such a range of services and variety of settings is not available, and that those services that are available and accessible do not respond adequately to the needs of carers or of the individuals being cared for. (However, most of the information is collected from the carers and does not therefore reflect sufficiently the views of the people with learning disabilities.) Armstrong (1989) reported that preferred provision would cover short periods during shopping hours, evening relief, overnight, weekends and longer periods of planned cover, as well as emergencies.

Scholl et al. (1991) surveyed seventy-eight carers in a study to determine their views of services provided. It was discovered that carers wanted services which covered part of the day and weekends, sitting services, play schemes and care in a family setting, rather than residential units or care in the client's own home. Many carers have expressed the wish for services to be local, flexible, easily arranged and immediately available (Ayer and Alaszewski 1984).

A report by the National Children's Home (1991) suggested that only 5 per cent of children with disabilities received short-term care services, and that over 50 per cent of families had no idea that short-term care was available. Scholl et al. (1991) discovered that 80–85 per cent of families were aware of relief outside of their own home, but that only 47 per cent were aware of relief within their own home. In addition to the findings that higher income groups and non-manual classes were more likely to receive short-term care, Stalker (1991) discovered that black and ethnic minority families were over-represented on waiting lists. It was also identified that the same groups figured highly among non-users who lack information regarding services available, and that services were presently insufficiently culturally sensitive.

The Children Act of 1989 demands that the cultural needs of children are considered when placing them in care, and that local authorities publish information about services more widely and in different languages. The problem of lack of knowledge regarding services is one which would be relatively easy to correct. However, if such services were widely advertised, then the demand for them may increase enormously. Services are poorly resourced, particularly in relation to family placement schemes. Here there is a need to cover payments to the respite carers, their training, travel expenses, any equipment required, the salary of staff employed to organise the scheme as well as office expenses. Robinson *et al.* (1991) surveyed the schemes available in the UK and found that virtually all had waiting lists, not always due to under-resourcing, but often to factors related to the person to be cared for, such as challenging behaviours, profound disability or even incontinence. (This reflects again the findings of Hubert (1991), who identified that the only form of short-term care generally open to this group of people is that in institutional settings.)

The solution to the problem of the under-funding may well be that individuals will be expected to cover the cost themselves. The National Health Service and Community Care Act 1990 has made provision for local authorities to charge for such services, and since there has been no financial help offered to assist in provision, any increase or improvement in services may be dependent on this course of action. Table 1.2 provides a summary of the social policy influences on short-term care.

Table 1.2 Policy influencing short-term care provision

Instrument	Policy
1952 DHSS Circ. 5/52	Officially recognises short-term care and recommends this form of provision.
1959 Mental Health Act	Informal admission to hospitals permitted, allowing the development of short-term services.
1970 Education Act	Daily attendance for children at school means more are able to live at home, increasing the potential demand for short-term care.
1971 White Paper	Places to be provided in existing homes, with foster parents/guesthouse proprietors.
1977 NDG Report No. 4	Short-term care for relief, assessment and treatment; recommends places within residential units, maintaining professionalism.
1978 Warnock Report	Recommends short-term care in a variety of forms.
1979 Jay Report	Recommends short-term care in wide-ranging forms.
1989 White Paper	Recommends a wide range of services, but sees short-term care as alternative accommodation.
1990 NHS and Community Care Act	Provides for charging people for the service.

Progress?

Despite the rhetoric of recent reports and recommendations, demand for short-term care is not being adequately met by statutory agencies, voluntary organisations or relatives and friends (Mitchell 1990). While it should not be encouraged more than necessary, there is evidence to support the idea that there is not enough in terms of quality, variety or availability for those people who require the service. The actual provision is disparate, largely unco-ordinated and inadequately documented, with little research or reference to service users. The variety of different agencies can cause confusion and difficulties in finding information, contacting the right person or gaining access, due to the demand (Oswin 1984, Ayer and Alaszewski 1984, Robinson *et al.* 1991, Scholl *et al.* 1991, Stalker 1991). Both Oswin (1984) and Hubert (1991) discovered that even when care was available, the quality of physical and emotional care was frequently inadequate, in that people were thought to be ignored for long periods. The cause of such conditions lies in a system which allows short-term care to be underfunded to the extent that the service is either non-existent or totally inadequate for some people.

The National Development Group (1977a) found that the value of short-term care is out of proportion to the amount of investment required. They also reported that the extent to which short-term care can be tailored to meet the specific needs of the individual will depend to some extent on the nature of those needs and also on the availability of resources, time, facilities and skill. Nearly ten years later the DHSS published a report which reviewed progress made in service for people with learning disabilities since the publication of the 1971 report (DHSS 1980). This report declared that agencies were fully stretched, and had to decide priorities among many competing claims. As a result, where there was already an existing service, the area would not be seen as a priority for short-term care. The implication for people with learning disabilities was that if the service they were receiving was a poor service, then this was the only one they were likely to get.

It is a poor reflection on 'progress' that there have been many policy documents produced, but few significant changes in practice. Those changes that have taken place are often due to creative individuals, usually parents or voluntary workers, who have put pressure on local authorities to provide contributions towards the costs of their schemes. It may be true that the finance available does not come from a bottomless pit, but it is also significant that a government, which emphasises the importance of such a service for all carers, appears to be unwilling to finance the development of the service.

SUMMARY

In an effort to maintain those features which are good about services provided for people with learning disabilities, there is a tendency to maintain other features which require drastic attention. Government policy is consistently recommending minor changes to the provision of services, but always with the accompanying reminder that changes must occur within the allocated resources. While it is claimed that spending on such services has been increased each year, these increases are generally the result of inflation and the expanding numbers of people requiring services, rather than improved provision. This leaves the onus for improvement on the service providers, who frequently come under considerable pressure from rising demands and falling services. Provision is therefore aimed at short-term crises rather than long-term needs. The result of this situation is that the staff working with the people with learning disabilities are left to 'get on with it'. They are expected to provide the best possible service within the options of their community, and to question the adequacy of those options in order to obtain additions to them (Durrant 1981).

Staff within the services frequently question the adequacy of such options, but resources are not forthcoming. However, perhaps it would not suit staff to protest too much either. Recommending too strongly that other options would serve the needs of people better may work towards the demise of their own role. Durrant (1981) suggests that time is short for professionals, who need to learn from their mistakes. If the staff of services, the family and carers and the people with learning disabilities could join forces and agree on the way forward, the policy-makers might find it more difficult to produce one face-lift after another (which only serves to give the illusion of improving services without achieving any real change).

Could there be a real collusion to maintain the status quo? The latest government guidelines identify ten areas of need for people with learning disabilities, but continue to appoint local authorities to ensure that these needs are satisfied. The difficulty here, of course, is that the local authorities are also responsible for defining those needs.

People with learning disabilities and their advocates must look elsewhere if they are hoping for any real change. If they wait for the services to undergo a metamorphosis, then it will be too late.

CASE STUDY

Jonathan is 19 years old. He is about to leave school and would like a job cleaning cars. He lives at home with his parents, an older brother and a sister who is 16 years old. Jonathan's brother, Andrew, is 22 years old and works as a mechanic in a large garage in the town. His sister, Mary, is still at school. The family live in a three-bedroomed terraced house. Jonathan's father, Mr Clarke, works as a baker. This means that he has to be at work by 4 a.m. Consequently he retires to bed early in the evening and is usually in bed by 9 p.m. Mrs Clarke works part-time in the local newsagent's. She works from 9.30 a.m. to 2 p.m. These hours have suited the family as she has always been at home to ensure that the children went to school and she was always there on their return.

Mr and Mrs Clarke know that Jonathan will attend the local ATC when he leaves school. They know that he wants to earn a living cleaning cars, but feel that he is being unrealistic. Mrs Clarke feels that if it was not for her efforts to get him out of bed in the morning, he would stay there all day. Jonathan is also said to have violent outbursts and frequent arguments with his father. The arguments usually centre around Jonathan playing his music after his father has gone to bed. His father complains that he plays it too loudly and that he cannot get to sleep. Jonathan and his sister also argue and Mary no longer brings her friends home because of this. Mary feels that as Jonathan does not have any friends himself, he is jealous of her friends and consequently embarrasses her in front of them. Mr and Mrs Clarke feel that the family needs frequent periods of time without Jonathan and arrange for Jonathan to receive short-term care in a local residential unit. Jonathan is said to be disruptive there. He does not like being there and thinks that his parents send him there because he argues with his father. He thinks that his parents do not want him any longer. While he is in the residential unit, Jonathan spends most of his time by himself and is bored.

Analysis

The issue of consumerism in relation to providing services to meet service users' wants is readily highlighted in this case study. Jonathan has clearly expressed his wish to earn his living washing cars. However, this choice is not responded to by either service providers or his parents. Instead, Jonathan, as with many other individuals with a learning disability, has to fit into the current pattern of service delivery. If a diversity of service provision existed, Jonathan would have an improved chance of actually being able to receive the type of service he wished. In addition to this Jonathan receives short-term care in an environment in which he is not happy. This reinforces the issue that in this instance it is the parents' needs that are being met, possibly to the detriment of Jonathan's well-being. The issue of who is the consumer is significant in this example as it would appear that the only person's needs not being met is the person with a learning disability, despite the fact that the services are supposedly in existence to meet such a person's needs.

KEY POINTS

Day service provision	Service provision
Defining need	Short-term care provision
Education	Social policy
Jay Report	The role of social services
Responsibilities of local	departments
authorities	Training centres

REFERENCES

Allen, D. (1990) 'Evaluation of a community-based day service for people with profound mental handicap and additional special needs', *Mental Handicap Research* 3 (2): 179–95.

Anderson, D. (1982) *Social Work and Mental Handicap*, London: Macmillan.

Armstrong, G. (1989) 'Family placement schemes', in N. Malin (ed.) *Reassessing Community Care*, London: Routledge.

Ayer, S. and Alaszewski, A. (1984) *Community Care and the Mentally Handicapped: Services for Mothers and their Mentally Handicapped Children*, London: Croom Helm.

Baldwin, S. (1991) 'From community to neighbourhood', in S. Baldwin and J. Hattersley (eds) *Mental Handicap Social Science Perspectives*, London: Routledge.

Blunden, R. (1991) 'Changing service systems: a contribution from research', in S. Baldwin and J. Hattersley (eds) *Mental Handicap Social Science Perspectives*, London: Routledge.

Carter, J. (1981) *Day Services for Adults (Somewhere to Go)*, London: George Allen and Unwin.

Department of Education and Science (DES) (1978) *Special Educational Needs: Report of the Committee of Enquiry of Handicapped Children and Young People* (Chairman Warnock), London: HMSO.

Department of Health (DoH) (1990) *The NHS and Community Care Act*, London: HMSO.

Department of Health and Social Services (DHSS) (1959) *Mental Health Act*, London: HMSO.

DHSS (1971) *Better Services for the Mentally Handicapped*, London: HMSO.

DHSS (1979) *Report of the Committee of Enquiry into Mental Handicap Nursing and Care*, London: HMSO.

DHSS (1980) *Mental Handicap: Progress, Problems and Priorities: A Review of Mental Handicap Services since the 1971 White Paper: Better Services for the Mentally Handicapped*, London: HMSO.

Duff, G. (1992) 'Respite choice', *Nursing Times* 88(33): 65–6.

Durrant, P. (1981) 'Personal social work', in A. Brechin, P. Liddiard and J. Swain (eds) *Handicap in a Social World*, Sevenoaks: Hodder and Stoughton.

Durrant, P. (1989) 'All in a day's service', *Social Work Today* 21(7): 15–17.

Goffman, E. (1961) *Asylums: Essays on the Social Situation of Mental Patients and Other Inmates*, Harmondsworth: Penguin.

Great Britain (1952) 'Short term care of mental defectives in cases of urgency', Ministry of Health Circular 5/52, in M. Oswin (1984) *They Keep Going Away*, London: King Edward's Hospital Fund.

Great Britain (1968) *Report of the Committee on Local Authority and Allied Social Services (Seebohm)*, London: HMSO.

Great Britain (1979) *Report of the Committee of Enquiry into Mental Handicap Nursing and Care*, vol. 1, London: HMSO.

Great Britain (1989) *Caring for People: Community Care in the Next Decade and Beyond*, London: HMSO.

Hancock, R. (1988) 'Developing day services' in D. Sines (ed.) *Towards Integration-comprehensive Services for People with Mental Handicaps*, London: Harper & Row.

Harper, G. (1989) 'Making each day matter', *Community Living* 3(1): 11.

Hattersley, J. (1991) 'The future of normalisation', in S. Baldwin and J. Hattersley (eds) *Mental Handicap Social Science Perspectives*, London: Routledge.

Hubert, J. (1991) *Home-bound*, London: King's Fund Centre.

Jahoda, A., Cattermole, M. and Markove, A. (1989) 'Day services for people with mental handicaps – a purpose in life?' *Mental Handicap* 17(4): 136–9.

King's Fund (1980) *An Ordinary Life: Comprehensive Locally Based Residential Services for Mentally Handicapped People*, London: King's Fund Centre.

King's Fund (1984) *An Ordinary Working Life: Vocational Services for People with Mental Handicap*, London: King's Fund.

Macdonald, I. (1991) 'Service for whom?' in S. Baldwin and J. Hattersley (eds) *Mental Handicap Social Science Perspectives*, London: Routledge.

McKnight, J. (1981) 'Professionalised service and disabling help' in A. Brechin, P. Liddiard and J. Swain (eds) *Handicap in a Social World*, Sevenoaks: Hodder & Stoughton.

MENCAP (1985) *Day Services Today and Tomorrow: Mencap's Vision of Daytime Services for People with a Mental Handicap*, London: Mencap.

Ministry of Health (1968) *Local Authority Training Centres for Mentally Handicapped Adults: Model of Good Practice*, London: HMSO.

Mitchell, F. (1990) 'Respite care services for adults: a survey of carers' views', *Mental Handicap* 18(10): 33–4.

Mooney, G. (1992) *Economics, Medicine and Health Care*, 2nd edn, London: Harvester Wheatsheaf.

Mooney, G., Russell, E. and Weir, F. (1986) *Choices for Health Care. A Practical Introduction to the Economics of Health Production*, 2nd edn, Basingstoke: Macmillan.

National Children's Home (1991) *Sharing the Caring – Respite Care for Children and Families*, London: NCH.

National Development Group for the Mentally Handicapped (NDG) (1977a) *Residential Short Term Care for Mentally Handicapped People: Suggestions for Action*, London: NDGMH.

NDG (1977b) *Day Services for Mentally Handicapped Adults*, London: NDGMH.

Nelson, S. (1989) 'Happier days', *Community Care* 19 Oct: 12–13.

Oswin, M. (1984) *They Keep Going Away*, London: King Edward's Hospital Fund.

Robinson, C., Orlik, C. and Russell, O. (1991) 'Someone to turn to', *Community Care* 2 May: 24–5.

Royal College of Nursing (1988) *The Health Challenge*, London: Royal College of Nursing.

Schneider, J. (1990) 'Care not custody', *Community Care* 6 Sept: 18–20.

Scholl, A., Saunders, M. and Radburn, J. (1991) 'Relief care for children and adults with a mental handicap', *Mental Handicap* 19(4): 161–4.

Seed, P. (1988) *Day Care at the Crossroads*, Tunbridge Wells: Costello.

Sloper, P. and Turner, S. (1992) 'Service needs of families', *Child Care Health and Development* 18(5): 259–82.

Social Services Inspectorate (1989) *Inspection of Day Services for People with a Mental Handicap*, London: HMSO.

Stalker, K. (1991) 'Missing out', *Social Work Today* 23(14): 29.

Teasdale, K. (1989) 'Day services', in N. Malin (ed.) *Reassessing Community Care*, London: Routledge.

Wolfensberger, W. (1972) *The Principle of Normalisation in Human Services*, Toronto: National Institute on Mental Retardation.

Chapter 2

Levels of intervention

Terri Lockyer and Tony Gilbert

INTRODUCTION

This chapter considers the contemporary debate concerning the efficiency and effectiveness of the practice of the two main professional groups working with people with learning disabilities and their families, that is, social workers and learning disability nurses. This debate has a long history and it has been productive in the sense that the examination of these two professions has led to both change and innovation. It is also true to say that it has led to a considerable amount of wasted energy. So why waste energy in either writing or reading this chapter?

The aim here is to provide a different way of looking at the debate and, for that matter, similar debates elsewhere. The intention is not to argue that one particular professional group should dominate the provision of support to learning disabled people. Rather, to propose that the different perspectives implicit within the practices of each profession can be seen to bring an additional richness to the care-planning process. These different perspectives can be defined in practice as different levels of intervention. In focusing upon these two professional groups there is a danger that the parts played by people with learning disabilities, their carers and other professional groups will appear to be marginalised. This is not the intention. However, to attempt to do justice to these other influences would be outside the scope of this chapter.

The identification of different levels of intervention provides a new focus for the debate over efficiency and effectiveness. This has usually taken place on the basis of seeking to identify tasks or skills of which either profession has a monopoly, or those that are shared between them. This type of debate tends to view skill as static, and it ignores the probability that either profession is perfectly capable of learning the skills of the other. In fact, both professions have had to learn many new skills since this debate began. The important distinctions, if there are any, lie within the processes of judgement and decision-making used by the respective professions. This is not to argue that these processes are not learned, as are the functional skills. Rather, it is to highlight that these 'ways of thinking' are formed in the process of socialisation into a profession. In this way, practitioners become the carriers of the profession's norms, values, beliefs and history. And it is in this that the understanding of its practice lies.

The format for the discussion in this chapter is set out in the following paragraphs. The first part of the chapter considers the historical development of the two professions. The aim is to focus upon the social and political context in which this development took place. This is in contrast to the rather sterile approach that presents social policy as a process of logical or evolutionary development. Policy does not develop in an ahistorical void, but is only made possible by the prevailing beliefs and values of the time. As a result certain things are only possible at certain times. In order to present this historical discussion it is necessary to take a broad-brush approach and a period of nearly 150 years is discussed in three relatively short sections. In doing this there is, of course, the danger of abbreviating history in such a way that it becomes distorted to meet the purposes of the analysis offered (Kumar 1978). However, the three sections have been chosen because they represent significant backgrounds against which the welfare state has been organised.

The first section considers the 'formative years' in the development of the professions from the mid-nineteenth century up to the formation of the welfare state. This was a period of *laissez faire* which also saw the great building programmes of asylums and colonies, as the 'insane' and 'feeble minded' were removed from urban areas and out of harm's way. The second section looks at the 'period of consensus' over welfare in the post-war years: a period in which Beveridge's report was implemented in order to end ill-health, poverty and squalor. At this time, Keynesian economics brought the belief that unemployment was a scourge of the past, and that careful management of the economy would pay for the welfare state. The final section considers the present environment, which is characterised by the breakdown of the post-war consensus.

The economic problems of the 1970s and the election in 1979 of a conservative government saw the beginning of a process of restructuring of the welfare state, leading to the present introduction of the National Health Service and Community Care Act (1990).

The second part of the chapter is set in the present and it focuses upon the concept of levels of intervention through the use of fictitious case studies. Here the aim is to demonstrate these levels of intervention in three different situations which might arise in community settings. In this it draws upon the principles in the Community Care Act of supporting informal care and consumer choice, and the targets set in 'Health of the Nation' (DoH 1991). The first case study considers the relationships between the primary healthcare team, community mental handicap nursing, and social work. The second case study considers the relationships between care management, community mental handicap nursing and social work. The final case study considers the relationship between psychiatry, community mental handicap nursing, and social work in the context of a specialist team for people who have offended.

LEARNING DISABILITY NURSING AND SOCIAL WORK: A HISTORICAL PERSPECTIVE

The formative years

The social and political context from which both the professions of social work and learning disability nursing have developed is that of the mid-nineteenth century and early twentieth century. It is important here to identify the dominant ideas and debates of this time, because they underpin the ways in which people then understood and discussed the social problems and issues they faced. These ideas set the frameworks within which the solutions were constructed. This period was dominated by a growing tension between the political and economic doctrine of *laissez faire*, and a recognition that there needed to be state intervention to control social unrest among the increasing numbers of urban poor.

There was also the issue of the general physical and mental fitness of the working class and its ability either to fight for the empire, or to provide the labour for Britain's economic success. The context was a rising level of international military and economic competition. Philanthropy was one response. Here a powerful moral doctrine, rooted in the Protestant work ethic, enabled the rich to provide assistance to the poor on condition that the recipients reciprocated by undertaking to improve their behaviour. The mere provision of assistance was viewed as morally dangerous, as it weakened the character of the recipient. The idea of 'self-help', which is still powerful today, is central to this doctrine.

The knowledge of people at this time was further informed by the emergence of an early understanding of genetics which, in turn, found its way into the social programmes advocated by the eugenics movement. This brought with it a new fear about the danger to society of 'hereditary pauperism' amongst the feeble-minded, which provided a focus for immorality, crime and disease. It also justified an increasing number of measures designed either to control or identify the mentally defective.

These concerns provided the background for two major developments in social policy. First was the continued development of the Poor Law, which, while it can be traced back to the times of Elizabeth I, underwent a rapid series of amendments throughout the nineteenth century. The growing fear of social unrest, culminating in the Swing riots of 1830, led to a Royal Commission report that resulted in the Poor Law Act of 1834. This act provided a landmark in terms of contemporary social policy in the distinction it drew between the 'deserving' and 'undeserving poor', categories which are still implicit within social welfare policy today,

> But more than just a means whereby the poor can be classified against some moral criteria as part of the social construction of welfare, the dichotomy symbolizes an important theme in the development of both social work and social security in Britain, even in the late twentieth century.
>
> (Ditch 1987: 24)

The second development in social policy was the increase in the number of asylums, set in motion by the County Asylum Act of 1808 and the Lunatics Act 1845. Specialisation within the Poor Law allowed for the recognition of a whole group of deserving poor, and it enabled those deemed to be suffering from 'unsound minds' to be moved from the workhouses and prisons to a place more suitable for their care (Carr *et al.* 1980). However, it was not until 1913 that a legal category of mental deficiency was established, with the passing of the Mental Deficiency Act. This caused a further specialisation within the state's provision and established the basis for the service that remains today.

The workhouse and the asylum provided the two main institutions of the late nineteenth- and early twentieth-century welfare state. The major difference was that the former sought to discipline the 'undeserving', while the latter disciplined the 'deserving'. It is to the gates of these institutions that the origins of both social work and learning disability nursing can be traced. However, while the role of social work developed in the social space between the institution and the community, because of the need to make judgements on the moral character of the poor and destitute, learning disability nursing had its origins within the asylum, where the inmates had already been defined as 'deserving'.

The development of social work in this space between the institution and society was also influenced by three other factors: a recognition that the institution did not provide the total answer, the need to make judgements about the 'deserving' and 'undeserving' poor, and the role of the Charity Organisation Society (COS). This latter organisation came into being in 1869 as a means through which the disparate philanthropic activity of that time could be organised and the threat of the 'clever pauper' tackled. The COS was 'committed to the application of rational and proto-scientific techniques to charity' (Ditch 1987: 26). In this it developed a number of workers who were to provide 'gatekeeping' roles to the means of support and assistance allowed by the Poor Law.

The COS was emphatic that the problems of poverty could not be alleviated by the mere giving of money, and that therefore self-help was a moral necessity. There was an elitist bias to this argument which the Webbs describe as an assumption that the rich were intellectually and morally superior to the poor (Webb and Webb 1929). The COS developed the casework model which is still prominent in social work practice today. Training in the casework method enabled the worker to visit people in their home circumstances, and to gather and document evidence from their family, friends and acquaintances as to their character. The 'deserving' were then helped through a series of structured and supportive visits which provided material assistance, on the basis that the recipients committed themselves to some form of moral improvement. The 'undeserving' were identified and passed on to the workhouse.

The influence of the COS declined in the early part of the twentieth century and its moral philosophy gave way to the new science of psychology, especially among those social workers working with people with learning disability (Clarke 1988a). What remained was the social worker's role in deciding whether an individual was deserving or not. Social work also became increasingly specialised, with social workers being employed in the hospital services, the prison and probation services, as well as in welfare. The association between social work and the Poor Law ended when the final elements of Poor Law legislation were repealed in 1948. However, the association between social work and the poor remains today (Becker and MacPherson 1986).

At the same time that training in social work practice was being developed through the COS, training was also being introduced for the attendants who worked in the asylums. The developing influence of the Eugenics movement, with its theme of the 'danger' posed to society by the unidentified imbecile and the link to hereditary pauperism, led to the creation in 1913 of a separate and segregated service for the mentally defective. The Royal Medico-Psychological Society (RMPA), which in 1890 began to provide the first uniform training for mental nurses (Carr *et al*. 1980), also took the lead in providing a similar training for people working with the mentally defective. This training focused upon anatomy and physiology, psychology, the nature of mental and moral deficiency, as well as the practices in physical nursing and the training of defectives. Such 'knowledge' also established the 'scientific' basis for paternalism within learning disability nursing, which then became fully integrated into the medical model as the relationship between mental deficiency and medicine developed.

Training through the RMPA continued up to the creation of the National Health Service in 1948 when the mental deficiency colonies, along with the asylums, were removed from local authority control and placed under the new Ministry of Health to become hospitals. In 1951 the register for mental nurses was created and within this there was a subsection for the names of nurses registered for the care of the mentally defective.

To summarise, it can be seen that the same social forces provided the motivation for the creation of both social work services and learning disability nursing. However, the role in social work of judging the 'deserving' originated from a moral ideology of self-help within the community. This was represented in the practice of casework. Within this was established a tradition which includes both the acceptance and rejection of particular cases. This is not the same for learning disability nursing, whose origins are in work with the 'deserving' poor. Decisions regarding eligibility are not therefore part of its history. In this profession, the influences of eugenics and medicine provided the basis for paternalism; the 'immoral' are incapable of self-control and therefore need to be controlled to protect both themselves and society.

The consensus years

The next period focused on in this discussion is that between the 1950s and the late 1970s, often referred to as a period of social and political consensus over the benefits and responsibilities of the welfare state (Gamble 1987). It was a period in which poverty and unemployment were seen to have been eradicated and the term 'the affluent society' was adopted. There was also a feeling that life was becoming more complex. It was a period of enlightenment when the two professions of learning disability nursing and social work enjoyed quite different fortunes.

The focus within welfare moved away from the morality of the poor to the idea that there were a few individuals and families who needed continuing support in order to survive in an increasingly complex world. There was also an increasing focus upon the way the fragmented nature of specialised services made it difficult to deliver or co-ordinate the complex packages of services that were often required.

> One study after another has shown that the personal social services devote most of their resources to a small proportion of their clientele, and many of these people need help from several different specialised services. Human needs do not come in self-contained specialised packages; they are entangled, involving whole families – and sometimes whole neighbourhoods.
>
> (Donnison *et al.* 1962: 2–3)

There was also a concern in social work to move away from being considered a service which dealt with problem families, to one which provided a service to anyone who wished to use it (Clarke 1988b).

It was against this kind of background that the Kilbrandon Committee report in 1964 (Scotland), and the Seebohm Committee report in 1968 (England and Wales), criticised the fragmented and patchy nature of social service provision. Their proposals were for the reorganisation of social services into single generic departments organised by the local authority. The Seebohm Committee argued for 'a new local authority department, providing a community based and family orientated service, which will be available to all. This new department will, we believe, reach far beyond the discovery and rescue of social casualties' (Seebohm Committee 1968 para. 2).

These new reorganised departments brought together a wide range of field work services that all tended to use the casework method of intervention. Also brought into these departments were a wide range of residential and day services catering for a diverse range of client groups, such as children, the elderly, the disabled and people with learning disabilities. This led to a continuing tension within social work between field and residential social workers. The residential workers included fewer professionally trained social workers, received lower salaries, and were generally considered as having a lower status than their field work colleagues. This division was highlighted by the existence of two different qualifications, the Certificate of Qualification in Social Work (CQSW), and the Certificate in Social Services (CSS), which tended to be held by field workers and residential workers respectively.

This period was also one in which a number of related issues came to bear upon the practice of institutionalisation. First, there was the increasing evidence from a number of quarters regarding the effects of institutionalisation and the dehumanising practices it encouraged (Barton 1959, Goffman 1961, King *et al.* 1971). Second, there was the long-standing problem of poor conditions in the mental handicap hospitals, which had been well known before the creation of the NHS: 'Bevan in 1950 warned his cabinet colleagues about the likelihood of scandal breaking out about the poor conditions in the mental hospitals' (Klein 1989: 80). Third, there was the resistance of the medical profession to the switching of finance into mental handicap hospitals (Ryan and Thomas 1980, Klein 1989). And finally, ministerial pressure for an independent inspectorate had been strongly resisted by the institutionalised interests of both civil servants and the medical profession (Ryan and Thomas 1980). These issues were brought to a head by the series of public scandals resulting from hospital inquiries which punctuated the 1970s. The first of these was promoted by the then Minister of Health, Richard Crossman, who seized upon the report of the inquiry at Ely Hospital in his struggle with the medical profession. By publishing the report in full he gained a lever which he then used to divert funds from the acute sector to set up an independent inspectorate, the Hospital Advisory Service (HAS) (Klein 1989).

This political spotlight upon mental handicap services, in particular the role of the NHS hospitals, sparked a number of government-sponsored initiatives such as 'Better Services for the Mentally Handicapped' (DHSS 1971), which considered the future direction of services, and The National Development Team, which had powers of inspection and standard setting. Inevitably the spotlight also fell upon those who worked in the institutions. And, while medical power and management indifference was criticised, it was learning disability nursing that found itself being scrutinised. This was partially as a result of moves to enhance the professional status of nursing in general.

The Briggs Report (DHSS 1972) proposed that learning disability nursing should be reorganised and that a new caring profession which was less medically orientated should emerge. The Jay Committee (DHSS 1979) was commissioned to consider this proposal in the light of other developments such as community care, and the increasing influence of 'normalisation' as an alternative to the medical model of care. There was also the need to consider the changes in the organisation and philosophy of the social services departments as a result of the Seebohm recommendations noted earlier. In the event, the committee's conclusion in respect of staff training was that this should become the responsibility of the training body for social work (CCETSW). This proposal, linking learning disability nursing with the low status 'Cinderella' services of residential social work, was met with considerable protest.

During this time there were also some interesting developments in the mechanisms through which social workers and learning disability nurses worked together. Primarily this resulted from the recommendations of The National Development Team (DHSS 1980), for the establishment of community mental handicap teams whose main role was to promote community services through finding practical solutions in the community to the problems faced by families. This brought a recognition of the developing role of the community mental handicap nurse (CMHN) who, in a similar way to the social worker, carried a caseload of clients and their families. However, the CMHNs did not carry the statutory powers of the social worker in respect of the Mental Health Act, child protection, or places of safety. What they did do was provide an example of practice outside of the residential setting which paralleled the practice of the field social worker. And, as in social work, these field practitioners were considered to be of a higher status than their residentially based colleagues.

To return to the concept of levels of intervention, the emergence of 'normalisation' as a service philosophy provides an interesting topic upon which to conclude the period of consensus. For it sat very differently within the values and beliefs of the two professions, with the most obvious tensions between the two surrounding the idea of choice. With respect to social work, normalisation appeared to fit easily with its traditional values of assistance on the condition of self-help. A social model committed to the prevailing norms of society provided a theoretical underpinning where the concept of choice could be used to answer any deviation from those norms. The original moral association between help and commitment to change behaviour was replaced by a humanistic notion of personal autonomy. This meant that there was no link between an individual's behaviour and the responsibility of a service or practitioner for that behaviour.

The concept of choice was more difficult to accommodate within the traditions of learning disability nursing. Here, the value base was developing out of the paternalism implicit within both the medical model and that of behavioural psychology, which was very influential in the 1970s. The idea of personal autonomy for the patient was attenuated by both a service and practitioner commitment to a duty of care, in which both accepted a responsibility for the actions of the person.

These different responses are reflected in the idea of different levels of intervention, for as stated earlier the different value bases of each profession influence the judgements and responses of the practitioner. This has led at times to tensions and misunderstandings between the professionals concerned. However, these differences can be considered as essential elements in the process of generating new possibilities for people with learning disabilities. The tensions between the different viewpoints need to be identified within a dialectical process in which new and often previously unthought-of possibilities can be generated from the resolution of conflicting positions. This is achieved through the development of a new position which accommodates the principles of the different viewpoints, while at the same time being more than just the mere sum of these principles.

The return of the market

The third part of this discussion of the historical development of learning disability nursing and social work considers the period from 1979 to the present. The election of the Conservative government in 1979 is seen to mark the end of the consensus which governed welfare politics in the post-war years. The reasons given for this breakdown differ depending upon which particular perspective you adopt. For the present it may be useful to identify some common elements within the social and political context of the 1980s.

The first surrounds the apparent failure of Keynesian economics to find solutions to the problems faced by Britain and the re-emergence of both poverty and unemployment. The second concerns the failure of the welfare state to meet the aspirations of all. Included within this is a growing voice of the users of services that seeks to challenge the institutional interests of welfare managers and professionals. The third focuses upon the apparent lack of morality in society with divorce, child abuse, civil unrest, violence and crime seemingly on the increase, and a breakdown of traditional values of respect and family life. For some the welfare state represents the case of this moral decline in that it has undermined personal responsibility and self-help (Davies 1987).

The political solution to many of these problems is seen to lie with social attitudes towards the welfare state. There is therefore seen to be a need:

1 To restructure the welfare state, withdrawing direct state provision, and to introduce market principles to discipline providers and to promote choice.
2 To re-establish morality in welfare provision, with a reinstatement of the philanthropic principles of assistance, with the reciprocal commitment from the recipients to change their behaviour. The social fund becomes a case in point.
3 To indentify the 'undeserving'; this can be seen in the growing antagonism towards universal benefits, the idea of the social security scrounger, and of the unemployed as partially consisting of the work-shy and those working in the 'black economy'.

It is against this background that contemporary community care policy operates. The family has been cited as having the major responsibility for care, with the idea of neighbourhood networks invoked to widen informal care to include neighbours, friends, and other relatives. However, there are growing concerns over the reality of this, both in its demands and in the way it falls disproportionately upon women (Ungerson 1987). The role of the state is to support and facilitate these networks of care. The NHS and Community Care Act (1990) restructures services in market terms of providers and purchasers, and it refers to consumers, choice and quality. It also identifies the role of the family and makes the support of informal carers one of its major objectives.

This restructuring, as with restructuring elsewhere, brings with it a declining role for both local government in making decisions over the services it provides, and for the local authority in the direct provision of care. Instead, the role of the local authority is defined as the assessment of individual needs and the purchasing of services from the private and voluntary sectors, or the NHS, to meet those needs. At the same time, the Health Service's role in community care is clearly in the provision of what are considered to be health needs, rather than social needs.

The central mechanism through which these needs are to be assessed, packages of care co-ordinated and evaluated, is that of 'care management'. Care management is tightly linked to budgetary limits with the aim of controlling the spiralling costs of welfare. It also challenges the institutionalised interests of professionals through a fragmentation of the professionals' ability to define both the need and the solution of that need. The care manager can commission an assessment from a range of providers, but the acceptance of its recommendations depends upon a negotiation between the client and the care manager, and upon the costs of the intervention. This is argued to introduce a meaningful set of choices for the consumer into care planning.

The professions of social work and learning disability nursing have had to respond in different ways to the demands of assessing social care and health care. The necessary definitions have been problematic, first in respect of being able to distinguish a health need from a social need, and second in respect of making this distinction with regard to individual people. The exact determination of such distinctions is a matter for local decision.

However, the basis for these definitions was set out by the Department of Health in 1991 by the then Health Minister Stephen Dorrell (H91/286). This circular refers to social care as the provision of a range of support which includes: accommodation,

activities of daily living, supporting personal and social relationships, developing socially competent behaviours, creating opportunities, using ordinary facilities, developing occupational skills
and supporting employment, facilitating health care and access to
other statutory services, counselling clients and informal carers
with respect to existing services, and the provision of social work
help to support emotional or practical stress. For social work the
'return to the market' marked an end to the Seebohm era's concept
of a universal service. But on the other hand, as a profession, it has
always operated in the environment of social needs, and the
decision-making over whether to respond to a particular need is
within its traditions.

Learning disability nursing finds itself in a more difficult
position for many of the activities identified as social needs are seen
by the profession as part and parcel of its role. The definition of
health care in the same circular focuses upon the following services:
alternatives to ordinary health services where these are unable to
meet the needs of people with learning disabilities, specialist mental
health services for people with severe psychiatric problems or
behavioural disturbances, and NHS residential services for the
small number of people with complex multiple needs such as severe
or profound learning disabilities with physical and sensory disabilities or psychiatric conditions.

One of the responses of the profession to this challenge is seen in
the concept of 'facility independence' proposed in the Cullen
Report (Cullen 1991). This, in principle, suggests that learning disability nursing should adopt a caseload approach making specific
health interventions with people with learning disabilities regardless
of where they happen to be living. A second set of concerns for
those working in a health care context are the targets set by *The
Health of the Nation*. These focus upon coronary heart disease and
stroke, cancers, mental illness, accidents, HIV/AIDS and sexual
health, and they involve issues such as exercise, diet, smoking and
safety.

CASE STUDIES

This next section develops the analysis of the different levels of
intervention through the use of three case studies. These are used to
demonstrate how different ways of approaching an issue generate
different possibilities for the person. This may arise because a

particular practitioner can enable access to different sorts of service, or to a specialist service. Alternatively, a different viewpoint may lead to a new way of thinking about an issue. In constructing these case studies the aim has not been to provide definitive examples of practice but to generate discussion.

Case study 1: the Griffin family

This first case study considers the relationship between the primary health care team, community mental handicap nursing and social work. The Griffin family live on a new, fairly exclusive housing estate on the edge of a major city. John and Rachael Griffin have three children. Mark, the eldest, is in his first year at university. Jennifer, who is 12 years old, is a bright and very independent young woman who aims for a career in science. Sarah, who is now 4, was born prematurely and has severe learning and physical disabilities. She is epileptic, and has ongoing medical needs resulting from congenital heart and lung abnormalities.

Sarah needs considerable attention, and is unable to walk and cannot sit up without support; she is also incontinent. However, from her family's viewpoint the most serious problems are with her eating, which results from the difficulties she has with swallowing due to her cerebral palsy. This means that she takes a very long time to have a meal and that she is prone to choking. Sarah also suffers from asthma. She is prone to acute attacks which usually means that she has to be hospitalised. These tend to leave Mrs Griffin emotionally and physically drained. There has always been considerable tension in the household but until recently this tension has generally been used in productive ways. However, fourteen months ago, Mr Griffin lost his job. Since then life for the Griffins has become increasingly difficult. Mrs Griffin wants help from her husband in caring for Sarah, something which he is increasingly reluctant to do.

The initial referral for Sarah came to the community mental handicap nurse (CMHN) from the primary health care team (PHCT) based at the local health centre. Until recently the family had been receiving specialist input from a community paediatric nurse who had been working to build up the family's confidence with respect to Sarah's asthma. Sarah also attends the health centre for physiotherapy sessions every other day and a fortnightly session with the speech therapist.

The reason for the referral was that it was hoped that Sarah would soon attend a pre-school group which would benefit both her and her mother. However, Mrs Griffin was reluctant for Sarah to go because of her concerns over her eating and asthma. Vicky Rogers, the CMHN, began her visits with the primary aim of encouraging Mrs Griffin to come to a point where she would feel able to leave Sarah at the group. She discussed this with Mrs Griffin and they drew up a plan where she would accompany Mrs Griffin and Sarah to the group and would then, over a period of time, support Mrs Griffin's withdrawal. Each visit to the playgroup would be followed up with a visit to Mrs Griffin to discuss her feelings and to evaluate progress.

In the process of visiting, Vicky became conscious of the anxiety in both Mrs Griffin and the other members of the family. She felt that this might be due to Sarah's eating problems. Therefore she began to work through in practice the advice that Mrs Griffin had been given by both the physiotherapist and the speech therapist. Unfortunately as Mrs Griffin had never been able to see both of them at the same time the advice had appeared to be contradictory. This had resulted in her adopting an *ad hoc* arrangement which left Sarah in a very bad sitting position and exacerbated her difficulties in swallowing. In working with Mrs Griffin and Sarah, Vicky was able to give some dietary advice which would help both Sarah's chewing action and her need for a balanced diet.

However, as she developed her intervention, Vicky became increasingly worried by the tension in the family and the way much of this was focused on Sarah. Vicky was worried that Sarah might be at risk from physical or emotional abuse. She therefore sought the advice of her CMHT colleague, Mary Summers, a social worker. In her discussions with Vicky, Mary sought to establish the basis for her concerns and whether she had any evidence to support these fears. In fact there was little evidence that abuse had ever occurred. However, Mary felt that the social stress the family was experiencing gave grounds for concern, and she decided to visit the family.

Mary and Vicky discussed which was the best approach, and while Vicky did not wish to disrupt her relationship with Mrs Griffin, Mary was clear that she had to act in Sarah's interests. On her next visit Vicky suggested to Mrs Griffin that the family might benefit from a contact with Mary Summers. At first Mrs Griffin was reluctant even to consider the idea. However she did eventually agree to Mary visiting, on the basis that she was Sarah's social worker. During this time Vicky reached a point where Sarah was attending the pre-school group and Mrs Griffin felt confident in leaving her there. She had done some training sessions with the staff with respect to what to do if Sarah had an asthma or epilepsy attack.

Mary had been able to visit the family on a number of occasions and she was able to discuss family issues with Mrs Griffin. Through this Mary had been able to assure herself that Sarah was not at risk. She was also able to help Mrs Griffin with a volunteer support worker from the local scheme she had organised. This worker would be able to provide two hours help per week. Mrs Griffin felt that this would be of most benefit if she could use this time to get some relief at mealtimes. This would mean that she could sit with the rest of the family and have her meal, something she rarely managed to do.

In summary, Vicky's original referral related to Sarah being able to access an ordinary playgroup facility. Here there were two interrelated issues: the first was to develop Mrs Griffin's confidence in order that she would be able to leave Sarah at the group; this would give her some respite from caring and it was hoped that it would be beneficial for her mental health. The second was to do with Sarah's development and having the opportunity to experience other children. In developing this intervention Vicky was able to identify the tensions within the family. She sought to tackle these on one level through working on Sarah's eating difficulties with her mother. This also enabled her to co-ordinate the advice of other health care professionals, and suggest ways of improving her diet. On another level Vicky sought the advice of her colleague Mary, who has responsibilities and powers under the Children's Act 1989, to ensure that Sarah was not at risk. However, in establishing contact with the family Mary was able to facilitate social care through the volunteer service.

Case study 2: the Barnes family

This case focuses upon a family who live in an area which has now reorganised towards a care management system. Bryan Morris was previously a social worker with the community mental handicap team but has recently taken up the post of care manager. Bryan knows the Barnes family well as they have been active members of his caseload on and off for many years. The family consists of Mrs Shelagh Barnes and Mr Roger Barnes, and their children Steven (23 years), Sharon (21 years), Teresa (20), James (10), Rodney (9), and Tina (3). They live in a four-bedroomed house on a large estate in a major city. Both Mr and Mrs Barnes have a mild learning disability, and all of the children are considered to have some degree of learning disability.

Steven and Sharon have a mild learning disability and they attend a day service some four miles away. Steven is a shy boy whose great interest is anything mechanical. Sharon, on the other hand, is more out-going. She has recently developed a sexual awareness which is worrying both her parents and the instructors. Teresa has a severe learning disability and cerebral palsy with marked choreo-athetoid movements. This makes it very difficult for her to sit, eat, work, etc. However, she is a very aware person, as well as being very demanding. Teresa's care takes a long time, and her incontinence creates a considerable amount of washing. A good deal of Teresa's personal care is given by Sharon, who also tends to take her out both in the evenings and at the weekend. This means that Teresa is quite involved in the activities that take place in the streets outside their home.

James and Rodney are both considered to have mild learning disabilities.

They attend their local junior school which has followed a policy of integrating children with special needs into mainstream classrooms. This has worked well for both of them as they are confident and enjoy learning. They also have a large number of friends, some of whom have a learning disability, while others do not. They all live and play in the same area. Tina is the baby of the family and is developing well, although she has been a little slow in achieving her milestones. She is now able to walk and can speak one or two words.

The family had not been active clients of a CMHT member for about three years. However, in the last month two referrals for the Barnes family have been placed, this time with Bryan as care manager. The first came from Mrs Barnes herself who is worried that Sharon might get pregnant and is looking for help in preventing this. The second was from the day service where Teresa attends, who feel that they are unable to meet her need due to the level of disability. Bryan decides to visit the family to make an initial assessment of their circumstances. Following this he commissions assessments from a number of services, one of which is from Clare Davis, the community mental handicap nurse (CHMN).

Bryan asked Clare to visit both Teresa and Sharon Barnes with a view to making an assessment of their nursing and related health needs. Bryan is also concerned about the degree of stress Mrs Barnes is under caring for the family and Teresa. He therefore asks John Simpson, a social worker, to make an assessment of the family's social care needs. Both Clare and John agree that they will provide a completed assessment in two weeks. At the same time Bryan commissions a physiotherapy assessment, and he asks two other day services and a voluntary sector home providing a respite service if they will submit some costings.

Clare's assessment with respect to Sharon focused upon her sexual health needs. Following discussions with Sharon it was established that there were three areas where she would like support. The first was in the use of tampons, the second was in the area of contraception, and the third was to do with personal relationships. Clare's assessment of Teresa focused upon two sets of needs. Here she felt that Teresa needed intensive help in managing her own continence and that she would benefit from getting some exercise such as swimming. Clare also felt that Teresa and Mrs Barnes would benefit from respite care.

John's assessment of the family's social care needs focused upon three areas. The first related to the older children. Mr and Mrs Barnes were wondering when Steven and Sharon would leave home and what options were open for them. The second related to the provision of respite care for Teresa. Here Mrs Barnes was not quite convinced that short periods of relief care would be of any great benefit. She felt that Teresa was hard work all the time and she had some relief from her care with the help Sharon gave. The third area in John's assessment concerned the use of a laundry service to take some of the household burden away from the family so that they would have some time for each other.

Bryan, as care manager, received the assessments and made an appointment to go to see Mr and Mrs Barnes and Teresa and Sharon to discuss the various possible care packages. In respect of Sharon, Bryan was concerned that the discussion with her parents should be reassuring but that the details remain confidential to Sharon. If she then chose to discuss these with her parents then that was her decision. With respect to Teresa this was more difficult as her needs and the needs of the family were so closely linked. Following these discussions, two care packages were agreed. The first package, concerning Sharon, was that Clare would work with her in the areas identified in the assessment.

The second package, concerning Teresa, was more complex. Mr and Mrs Barnes felt that they wanted to consider an alternative place for Teresa to live. However Teresa did not seem very keen on the idea and indicated that she wished to stay at home. Bryan suggested that he might be able to get some support for Mrs Barnes such as a laundry service and occasional help in the home. This did not get Mrs Barnes's agreement as she felt that she would rather do the dirty washing herself. Bryan felt that the best course here would be to leave the family to consider the options and they would meet again in two weeks. Mr Barnes suggested that John and Clare might also be there to help them sort things out. In the meantime, Clare was to begin to work with Sharon.

As Clare's assessment had focused closely upon Sharon's needs with regards to her sexual health, they began working together to develop an educational programme that would enable Sharon to gain confidence with respect to her sexuality. This involved issues to do with relationships, assertiveness, choice and control. At the same time it involved practical issues such as managing menstruation.

After two weeks the meeting regarding the needs of the Barnes family and Teresa reconvened. This time Clare and John were there, and after considerable discussion they put together a package. This involved Teresa attending a day service managed by a cerebral palsy organisation. However, during the week she would live away from home, returning on Friday evenings. The place where Teresa would be living during the week was quite happy about the arrangement so long as there was some initial staff support with respect to Teresa's needs. Bryan asked Clare if she would make arrangements to provide these support sessions.

In summary, the needs of this family were complex as the needs of a particular member were not totally complementary to the needs of the other members. Bryan as care manager was responsible for putting together a package of support for both the individual members and the family. Sharon's needs could be met by Clare working from a health care perspective. However, with respect to Teresa, the views of the professionals

were rejected by either Mr and Mrs Barnes, or by Teresa. This demonstrates that professional definitions of need do not necessarily correspond
with needs as they are perceived by the users of services.

Case study 3: Michael Soames

Michael Soames is 46 years old, an able man with a mild learning disability
who is seeking to readjust to life back in his local community. Michael lives
in a small flat near the shopping centre where he remains subject to section
41 of the Mental Health Act 1983. Michael has had a long history of mental
health problems. He was diagnosed as schizophrenic at 17. He is also
epileptic and smokes heavily. The last two years of Michael's life have been
spent in the local mental handicap hospital. Previously he spent twenty
years in a special hospital. Michael moved into the flat about seven months
ago with high hopes that he would find a job and meet some new friends.
On the job front Michael is still attending the sheltered workshop where he
had been working as a carpenter for about eighteen months. However, his
attendance had recently become irregular.

Michael's support in the community comes from Nick Johns, a specialist
social worker, and Henry Phillips, the community mental handicap nurse.
They have been working with Michael ever since his arrival from the special
hospital. This referral was placed by Mary Roe, the consultant psychiatrist,
who is responsible to the Home Office for Michael's care and rehabilitation. Until a couple of months ago progress with Michael had been slow
but steady, and he had been motivated by the developments in his life.

However, life was not turning out to be all that Michael expected. Money
was tight, especially as he spent a good part of his wages on cigarettes. He
was lonely, and had no social life or other interests. He was also getting
careless with his medication and had recently suffered a number of
seizures. When Nick and Henry spoke to Michael he appeared depressed
and they felt that he was losing confidence in his ability to live on his own.
He saw his seizures as evidence that he was not being cared for properly.
Nick and Henry discussed their concerns with Mary Roe, who decided that
she would raise these with Michael at their next meeting. These are held on
a fortnightly basis. In the meantime Nick and Henry were asked to see
Michael and undertake an assessment of needs, focusing upon aspects of
residence, employment and leisure.

Nick, from a social work perspective, undertook with Michael an assessment which considered elements relating to social care. These included
issues relating to his benefits and his level of entitlement, the progress with
respect to his living circumstances, and his work situation. The main issue
for Nick was Michael's loneliness which he felt was at the base of most of
his present problems.

Henry, from a nursing perspective, provided a different focus upon issues relating to Michael's living environment, work and leisure. Henry looked, with Michael, at issues in the context of health gain and health loss. Henry felt that Michael's budgeting skills had slipped, he was buying food as he felt hungry, which usually meant that he would buy a pie or some chips. Also his expenditure on cigarettes was such that he would run out of money some time before his wages were due. Henry felt that these factors had contributed to a breakdown of any clear routine in Michael's life, a consequence of which was that his control over his medication had been lost. With respect to Michael's loneliness, Henry agreed with Nick that this was a major factor in his life.

Michael and Henry agreed that they would work on his budgeting, diet, and medication. Central to this would be an attempt to encourage Michael to cut down or stop smoking. This would benefit his health and give him more money for other things. They also agreed that they would start the process by looking at how Michael organised his money and household shopping. Henry agreed to call on the evening Michael was paid, to support him while he made a list of his household needs for the week, and then he would accompany Michael shopping. They could then reflect upon this over a drink in the pub.

With regard to Michael's difficulties with his medication, Mary agreed that she would discuss the issue with the local pharmacist so that Michael could pick up his medication weekly in a dispenser designed to identify the individual doses for each day. Henry would be responsible for monitoring this process.

There remained the major issue of supporting Michael in the development of personal relationships. This, they all agreed, was very important to Michael. However, they felt that they needed to be very careful not to provide the impression that they would be able to produce personal relationships. Rather, they saw it as essential that Michael was aware of the outcomes in respect of the interventions they aimed to carry out. Here they agreed with Michael that they would seek to promote opportunities. The first point that Michael made was that if he had a 'real job' then he would have a better chance of meeting some friends. They all agreed that this was a good point and that Nick would look into the possibilities of a new job. But the point was also made that Michael would need to be fit and organised if he was to be successful in this aim.

Nick suggested that he would work with Michael on his inter-personal skills as these are essential to developing his social care. Here he suggested to Michael that he might like to join a men's group that he had helped set up, and Nick offered to accompany Michael for the first few occasions. Henry was also committed to supporting Michael in establishing personal and social relationships as he saw these as important to Michael's mental health. He suggested to Michael that they could go to the local bingo hall once a week. Michael welcomed the suggestion as he liked to do something when he was out, rather than just sit in the pub drinking. Henry felt that this would provide an opportunity for Michael to meet people. It would also provide a further focus for Michael's budgeting as he would need some money with which to go out, and it might therefore motivate him to stop smoking.

In summary, it can be seen that Michael's health needs are the primary factor in determining interventions for both social and health care. It can also be seen that a particular need, in this case personal relationships, can be approached from both a health care and a social care perspective. Here the rationale for the intervention and the criteria against which it is evaluated, i.e. health gain or health loss, will differ. However, each intervention is complementary to the other, and both hold the potential for a positive outcome for Michael.

SUMMARY

This chapter has tried to identify the contributions of two professions, social work and learning disability nursing, to the care of people with learning disabilities in the context of the idea of different levels of intervention. Each profession brings a different perspective to the support of such people in community settings. A focus on their development showed how each profession came to carry distinct beliefs, values, and histories and how this related to social and political welfare issues of concern at particular times. Inevitably in such a condensed history certain events are left out, for example, the detailed development of community care policy and the changing emphasis within its applications; the process of de-institutionalisation; and the contemporary pressure upon social work arising from concerns over child care practices. However, even from a brief account it can be seen how the different perspectives of each profession has developed and how this can contribute to the richness of opportunities for improved support of people with learning disabilities.

Contemporary welfare is dominated by the restructuring brought about by the introduction of the NHS and Community Care Act, and the distinctions resulting from the idea that social care can be clearly separated from health care. The implications of this are different for the respective professions. Learning disability nursing is seeking to identify its practice in the context of health needs, a notion with which it has enjoyed an ambiguous relationship since the late 1960s. Social work, on the other hand, appears to be returning to its traditional 'gatekeeping' activity in respect of welfare services.

Three case studies have been used in an attempt to demonstrate the way in which these issues might become apparent in contemporary practice. They also demonstrate the types of relationships that might be structured between different professionals and the recipients of their service. It is hoped that the concept of different levels of intervention can provide the basis for a more productive debate than the one conducted up to now about the contributions that different professionals make to the lives of people with learning disabilities.

KEY POINTS

Care management

Choice

Community care

Consensus years

Deserving and undeserving poor

Health care

Institutionalisation

Marginalisation

Paternalism

Professionalism

Social care

Social policy

Welfare state

REFERENCES

Barton, R. (1959) *Institutional Neurosis*, Bristol: Wright.

Becker, S. and MacPherson, S. (1986) *Poor Clients*, Nottingham: Benefits Research Unit, Department of Social Administration, University of Nottingham.

Carr, P., Butterworth, C. and Hodges, B. (1980) *Community Psychiatric Nursing: Caring for the Mentally Ill and Handicapped in the Community*, Edinburgh: Churchill Livingstone.

Clarke, J. (1988a) *Social Work: The Personal and The Political, Unit 13 Social Problems and Social Welfare*, Milton Keynes: The Open University.

Clarke, J. (1988b) *Social Work in the Welfare State, Unit 14 Social Problems and Social Welfare*, Milton Keynes: The Open University.

Cullen, C. (1991) *Caring for People: Community Care in the Next Decade and Beyond. A Report to the Four Chief Nursing Officers*, London: HMSO.

Davies, C. (1987) 'Towards the remoralization of society', in M. Loney, R. Bocock, J. Clarke, A. Cochrane, P. Graham and M. Wilson (1987) *The State or the Market: Politics and Welfare in Contemporary Britain*, London: Sage.

Department of Health (DoH) (1989) *The Children Act: An Introductory Guide for the NHS*, Manchester: Health Publications Unit.

DoH (1990) *The National Health Service and Community Care Act*, London: HMSO.

DoH (1991) *Guidance on Facilities for People with Learning Disabilities, H91/286*, Press Release, 25.6.91, London.

DoH (1991) *The Health of the Nation*, Cmnd 1523, London: HMSO.

Department of Health and Social Security (DHSS) (1971) *Better Services for the Mentally Handicapped*, Cmnd 4683, London: HMSO.

DHSS (1972) *Report of the Committee on Nursing*, Cmnd 5115, London: HMSO.

DHSS (1979) *Report of the Committee of Enquiry into Mental Handicap Nursing and Care*, HN (79) 27 Cmnd 7468, London: HMSO.

DHSS (1980) *Development Team for the Mentally Handicapped, second report 1978-79*, London: HMSO.

Ditch, J. (1987) 'The undeserving poor', in M. Loney, R. Bocock, J. Clarke, A. Cochrane, P. Graham and M. Wilson (1991) *The State or the Market: Politics and Welfare in Contemporary Britain*, 2nd edn, London: Sage.

Donnison, D., Jay, P. and Stewart, M. (1962) *The Ingleby Report: Three Critical Essays*, Fabian Pamphlet, London: Fabian Society.

Gamble, A. (1987) 'The weakening of social democracy', in M. Loney, R. Bocock, J. Clarke, A. Cochrane, P. Graham and M. Wilson (1991) *The State or the Market: Politics and Welfare in Contemporary Britain*, 2nd edn, London: Sage.

Goffman, E. (1961) *Asylums: Essays on the Social Situation of Mental Patients and Other Inmates*, Harmondsworth: Penguin.

Gostin, L. (1983) *A Practical Guide to Mental Health Law: The Mental Health Act 1983 and Related Legislation*, London: Mind.

King, R.D., Raynes, N.V. and Tizard, J. (1971) *Pattern of Residential Services for Mentally Handicapped Children*, London: Campaign for the Mentally Handicapped.

Klein, R. (1989) *The Politics of the NHS*, 2nd edn, London: Longman.

Kumar, K. (1978) *Prophecy and Progress: The Sociology of Industrial and Post-industrial Society*, Harmondsworth: Penguin.

Ryan, J. and Thomas, F. (1980) *The Politics of Mental Handicap*, Harmondsworth: Penguin.

Seebohm Committee (1968) *Report of the Committee on Local Authority and Allied Personal Social Services*, Cmnd 3703, London: HMSO.

Ungerson, C. (1987) *Policy is Personal: Sex, Gender and Informal Care*, London: Tavistock.

Webb, S. and Webb, B. (1929) *English Poor Law History: Part Two: The Last Hundred Years*, vol. 1, London: Longman.

Part II

Judgement, decision-making and practice

The first part of the book has discussed issues which arise from the development and implementation of policy decisions. The second part now develops the discussion by considering the implications for practice of two key concepts. These two concepts, choice and empowerment, are often referred to in the debate over what services and professional practice should aim to achieve. However, before entering the debate, Chapter 3 sets out the problematic nature of judgement and decision-making within human services. It focuses upon ethical theories and the resulting codes of behaviour developed to guide practice, against which judgements are compared.

In beginning the discussion with a focus on ethics the intention is to make the connection between what a society expects of its professional practitioners on the one hand, and on the other the everyday decisions they make. Decision-making is not, and cannot, be left to the arbitrary whims of individual professionals. The status of the professional is one that brings with it the requirement both to exercise judgement and to subject that judgement to the scrutiny of others. These others might be the users of a particular service, one's own peers, or the providers of a service. In some circumstances professional workers may be called to justify their actions within a legal process, or they may have to justify them to the state itself.

Ethical theory, it will be argued, provides professional practice with the basis for decision-making. However, a knowledge of ethics will not remove the need to exercise judgement, for professional practice requires that decisions are made which take into consideration the complexity of the circumstances in which humans live their lives. Rather, from ethics we derive a series of codes, or principles, through which professional judgement can be applied and explained. In turn, this provides a means by which society can pass its judgement upon the activities and practice of particular professionals, or groups of professionals.

Following on the discussion of ethics Chapter 4 provides an analysis of the concept of informed choice. Choice is an often used but seldom explained idea within human services. This chapter aims to clarify the basis upon which a choice can be considered to be either informed or not informed. In doing this it also identifies the implications of choice for professional practice, and the responsibilities professionals have in promoting informed choices among their clients. Again, the issue of judgement is essential to the process of securing informed choice. Practice which excludes choice or frustrates choice can be considered as paternalistic, dependency creating, and unethical. On the other hand, choices which are exercised on the basis of ill-informed judgement can be considered to be negligent.

Chapter 5 considers the idea of empowerment, often claimed to inform contemporary services. This chapter reveals the complex and ambiguous nature of the concept and analyses it within the context of professional practice. This is developed through a discussion of practical strategies aimed at achieving empowerment, which, in turn, raise issues for practice. This chapter identifies some of the ethical considerations that are necessary when working in empowering ways.

Chapter 3

Ethical issues

Margaret Todd

INTRODUCTION

The aim of this chapter is to identify the importance of judgement in everyday practice. In this context, judgement will be related to those complex decisions practitioners often face that present them with a moral dilemma. The resolution of moral dilemmas lies within the realm of ethics. The two main theories of ethics which underpin decision-making in the context of care will be explained and their implications discussed. These theories, utilitarianism and deontology, rest upon different propositions and therefore the implications for the client, their carers and professional practitioners may differ depending upon which perspective is applied. Briefly, the main tenet of the utilitarian perspective is to promote the greatest good for the greatest number of people. Thus the consequences of actions are of over-riding concern. In contrast, the deontological perspective holds that some actions are right in themselves, regardless of the consequences, and that the rights of the person, that is their human rights, are of primary importance.

However, before moving on to discuss these particular perspectives it is necessary to consider what ethics is. Essentially, while morality, or morals, refers to the standards of behaviour against which the acts of individuals or groups are judged, ethics refers to the study of such standards. In considering whether or not the act of a person in a particular context is morally right and ethically correct there are two levels of judgement. At the first level the act of the individual or group is considered in relation to a moral code. Different individuals or groups may follow different but equally convincing moral codes. For example, issues of abortion, divorce, and pre-marital sexual intercourse are considered differently depending upon moral conviction. At the second level, that of ethics, a generalisation is made, setting the different moral positions into an overarching debate about what should motivate human behaviour and how that behaviour should be judged. Here again there are different positions to be held, for example utilitarianism or deontology. The implications of this are that a particular society may judge an act to be ethical which a particular group in that society, possibly on religious grounds, considers immoral. It is in the attempt to provide guidance upon these issues that professional bodies, health care organisations, and social care organisations develop ethical codes of conduct and set up ethical committees to monitor the developing context of practice.

The objective of this chapter is to consider the influence the theories of ethics have upon practice. First it identifies the import-ance of human rights to the discussion and the effect this has on judgements. The next section then outlines the two broad ethical perspectives which tend to dominate the care environment, and their main tenets. This is followed by a section which looks briefly at ethical issues concerning the use of behavioural interventions. The final section examines the different models which have been developed to aid ethical decision-making and a fictitious case study is used to highlight some of the tensions between different ethical perspectives.

HUMAN RIGHTS

Before considering ethical theories it is useful to consider the issue of human rights, as these need to be promoted when making decisions of an ethical nature. The United Kingdom signed the United Nations Declaration of Human Rights in 1948. Broadly speaking, these rights are in relation to individual freedoms and the responsibilities accorded to them. This idea of associated responsi-bility is important as it sets constraints to the right of personal freedom which should be exercised in such a way that it does not impede the freedoms of others. Osmanczyk (1985) outlines some of the basic rights of individuals, summarised as follows:

1 All human beings are born free and equal.
2 The rights and freedoms apply to everyone without discrimina-tion on any grounds.
3 Everyone has the right to life.

4 Everyone has the right to own property.
5 Everyone has the right to freedom of thought, opinion and expression of these opinions.

In the United Kingdom a problem arises because although we have signed the United Nations Declaration, the rights enshrined in it have no legal status. Thus, minority groups such as people with a learning disability may find that the exercise of their rights is subordinated to the exercise of the rights of the majority. In addition to these basic human rights the government has afforded individuals other rights, in particular those that relate to health and social care, and public services. These rights are outlined in the Patient's Charter, the NHS and Community Care Act (1990), and the Citizen's Charter respectively. However, again, some of these rights do not have the force of statute and therefore the individual has not got the right to legal redress if these are denied.

Conflicts and tensions can and have arisen when individuals with a learning disability have attempted to uphold their rights. Moreover, many people with a learning disability rely upon others – relatives, carers, advocates – to safeguard their rights. This gives rise to tensions between care workers, other professionals and service providers. Such tensions can be so severe that they cause other relationships between these individuals or agencies to break down. In respect of ethical decisions these tensions may be very severe; in fact some have to be resolved in settings such as the High Court, or the European Court. However, in most cases such decisions have to be reached, and are reached, in the local context of the people involved. This may result in decisions over rights that can be perceived as paternalistic and promoting dependence. This needs to be balanced against the consequences of the rights not being met.

The upholding of rights can also be problematic because the effect of applying a right may not have equal consequences for all those concerned. The declaration does not provide scope for determining whose rights take precedence in any given situation. An example to elaborate this issue may be useful. When several people with a learning disability reside in a 'group home', one of these individuals may wish to watch television, while another may wish to listen to compact discs on the music centre. The problem arises because both pieces of equipment are situated in the lounge, and the solution of rearranging the furniture so that both pieces of equipment are not in the same room is not possible. Therefore a conflict arises in relation to whose rights will be upheld and consequently whose rights will be sacrificed.

Carers and professionals face many similar tensions in their day-to-day practice and attempt to resolve them on the basis of fairness. This may involve negotiation; for example, the TV can be used this morning and the CD player this afternoon. Or, alternatively, it may mean that the situation is resolved through neither person having the opportunity. Either of these solutions can be considered unsatisfactory. Another, more effective, way of resolving these dilemmas is to utilise ethical theories to aid decision-making. These provide an established base upon which judgements can be made and against which they can be evaluated. Ethics are especially important to judgements made in the care sector as these have real and often complex consequences, which, in turn, hold both costs and benefits for all those concerned.

ETHICAL THEORIES

There are two main theories of ethics which are relevant to the discussion about judgements in caring situations. These have been identified as the deontological perspective and the utilitarian perspective (Block and Chadaff 1981). One view of the role of ethics is that it seeks to support the notion of the rights of the individual while establishing the corresponding duties of other people towards them. Rights and duties are thought of as absolutes in some sense. The difficulty with this notion is that it does not indicate whose rights should take precedence in a given situation. For example, how do you resolve the tension between a woman's right to have an abortion and the foetus's right to live (Hare 1991)? Thus it tells us little about how to decide what rights people have, other than those discussed in the earlier section. Or, if incompatible rights are claimed, it is not possible to say which ought to be given precedence, especially in circumstances where the consequences of a decision are absolute. This can be seen in the example above, where either the woman has the child or the foetus dies; there is no middle position which can be negotiated.

The utilitarian perspective

Teleology or consequentialism defines rights in terms of the good produced as the consequences of an action. Consequentialism holds that an act should only be judged right or wrong on the grounds of the consequences that are produced. Consequentialists would decide how they should act based on the likely outcomes of the action. The consequences will either be beneficial and therefore good, or disadvantageous and therefore bad, and this is predicted beforehand (Seedhouse 1992). Consequentialism is a global theory of ethics, and utilitarianism is a subset of this perspective.

Utilitarianism is classically associated with the goal of happiness or pleasure and with the writings of philosophers such as Aristotle (384–322 BC), Thomas Hobbes (1588–1679), Rousseau (1712–78), Jeremy Bentham (1748–1832), and most importantly John Stuart Mill (1806–73). This perspective does not depend upon duties or principles which are viewed to have the authority of command-ments. Nor does it assume that there is a naturally right thing to do. The motives behind actions are not considered to be the basis for the judgement of the act, rather it is the consequences of the act which are to be considered important. A basic tenet is that the person should always act to produce the greatest good over evil. The greatest good has historically been taken to mean the greatest happiness or pleasure for the greatest number of people. In order to determine if an action is good or bad a cost-benefit analysis must be made.

Here utilitarianism requires the decision-maker to be strictly impartial. That is, the person making the decision must consider him or herself as having equal importance and not more import-ance than all others concerned. This person should sacrifice self-interest if this will bring about the greatest good (Seedhouse 1992). However, if people make decisions based on the greatest good for themselves this would be egotism and ethically wrong. In utili-tarianism, the probable results of performing various actions relevant to a situation are calculated and the one chosen is that which is likely to produce more benefit than harm (Tschudin 1992). Actions that produce happiness are right and those that produce the opposite are wrong. Happiness is equated with pleasure and the absence of pain, while unhappiness is equated with pain and the privation of pleasure.

To summarise, the basic principle of utilitarianism is the greatest good for the greatest number. Actions are future-oriented and do not depend on historical duty (Tschudin 1992). The interests of all are of equal weight and decisions are made using cost-benefit analysis. While utilitarianism is one subset of consequentialism, it in turn contains a number of subsets. These are referred to as rule, act, and general utilitarianism. Each of these in turn places a different emphasis upon particular interpretations of promoting the greatest good. These are outlined below.

Act utilitarianism

Act utilitarianism states that in each situation the individual should ask, 'what effects will my actions have on the amount of good in the world?'. The individual taking the action needs to weigh up the benefits (good), and disadvantages (harm), of the actions. The decision over which act to follow should be based on creating more good. Therefore if the action produces more good than harm it should be done (Seedhouse 1992).

General utilitarianism contends that actions do not derive from unique responses to specific situations as act utilitarianism does, nor does it rely on rules. Rather it promotes the idea that any potential actors should ask themselves, 'What if everyone does what I propose to do?'. This places strong emphasis on the consequences of actions, the major tenet of consequentialism.

Rule utilitarianism

Rule utilitarianism, unlike general utilitarianism, stresses that the way to produce the greatest good in the long term is to keep certain rules. In fact obedience to these rules is fundamental to ethical decision-making. The aim of rule utilitarianism is to discover rules of conduct that produce the greatest good over evil. This involves a process of calculation, that is, rules can be discovered through rational human thought. The concept of rules here differs from that argued by deontologists who believe that rules exist prior to human experience. For utilitarians the justification of rules lies in their utility and not in their purity.

Health care workers currently work with rules that have been arrived at through a careful consideration of the consequences of actions, and the application of a cost-benefit analysis (Seedhouse 1992). Some professions, such as medicine and nursing, have professional codes of conduct which include ethical guidelines. These codes are specific rules that apply to the person in that profession and they are over and above the general moral codes which govern society as a whole. Professional codes provide action guidelines for the individual concerned. It is not possible for professional codes to incorporate all the moral principles on which they are based, as they would become too complex to aid decision-making. Consequently, codes of conduct alone may be insufficient to aid ethical decision-making but they certainly need to be taken into account (Beauchamp and Childress 1989).

The major problem which arises from the application of rule utilitarianism is that while it creates an excess of good over evil for the population as a whole, this good is not distributed fairly. A certain portion of the population may in fact suffer, but their suffering is outweighed by the gains made by the majority of the population. Thus the principle of justice is undermined by rule utilitarianism. Justice is seen as fairness, but involves contentious principles. The three types of justice are:

- To each according to his or her rights.
- To each according to what he or she deserves.
- To each according to his or her needs.

In the United Kingdom people have equal rights to own property. However, people with a learning disability rarely do own property and may find it difficult to obtain a mortgage, as do other groups excluded or marginalised in the employment market. Therefore inequalities exist. Similarly, it might be stated that people with learning disability deserve to own property in the same way as any other citizens, but most often they do not. In addition, the first two principles may undermine the third principle.

To reiterate, the main tenet of the utilitarian perspective is to seek the best consequences of actions. Morally right actions are those which are the most useful in producing the best consequences for everyone. Actions only have moral value if they are useful. Thus it is our moral obligation to try to produce the best consequences we can. These are summarised as follows.

1 The greatest amount of pleasure for the smallest amount of pain or suffering as possible.
2 The greatest amount of happiness and the least amount of unhappiness.
3 The greatest amount of human and animal well-being as possible.

Utilitarians accept that we cannot know if our actions do in fact produce the best consequences as we do not know what the consequences would be if we acted differently. However, we are morally motivated when we are concerned to make our actions as useful as possible in bringing about the best consequences. Insofar as moral motivation is concerned with the best consequences, morality itself cannot be seen to be its own reward. Rather, its value lies in the benefits it may produce (Rowson 1990). When people have a choice to make they have a moral obligation to look at all possible courses of action and assess the likely benefits, or otherwise, of each course of action for everyone involved. Greater benefits should be regarded as more valuable than smaller ones, and everyone should be regarded as equally important. This assessment should consider both the immediate and long-term benefits.

However, this approach is time-consuming and it may not be possible to follow it every time a decision is made; we need a rule of thumb about how to behave to which we can refer in a hurry. These rules are decided by working out which type of action would in most circumstances bring about the greatest benefit to everyone in the long term. It is thought that axioms such as 'keep your promises' or 'do not tell lies' are really utilitarian guidelines. These should be followed when we are in a hurry, but we do not have to stick to them when we have time to think things through (Rowson 1990).

The deontological perspective

Deontological theories oppose much that utilitarianism theories affirm. This perspective, most closely associated with H.A. Prichard and Immanuel Kant (1724–1804), maintains that obligation and right are independent of the concept of good. In contrast with utilitarianism, deontology holds that the right actions are not determined purely by good consequences. Thus it is believed that some features of acts other than their consequences make them either right or wrong. However, some acts are right or wrong because of right-making consequences such as fidelity to promises, truthfulness and justice (Beauchamp and Childress 1989).

Deontology, or non-consequentialism, defines right by considering features intrinsic to an action, for the most part independently of its consequences. Decisions about its rightness depend on the nature of the action itself. Deontologists are sceptical about the validity of predicting the consequences of an action and put a primary emphasis on the rights of the person, that is, human rights. Like utilitarianism, deontology also argues for the principle of justice. Within deontology a right action can only be considered to be such if it is done out of a sense of duty to a set of principles (Tschudin 1992). Thus, particular actions can be seen to be right or wrong in themselves. Morality is a matter of doing those actions which are right in themselves and avoiding those that are wrong in themselves.

The essence of ethics from a deontological perspective, therefore, is that people should act according to a set of principles which is their duty (Seedhouse 1992). This duty is pre-ordained and is not the result of a rational consideration of the possible consequences of the action. Certain duties are considered to be of supreme and abiding importance and should never be over-ruled. As with utilitarianism, there are different schools of thought within the deontological perspective. These are act and rule deontology, which will be considered below.

Act deontology

This is an extreme form of deontology in which the duties and principles are not defined beforehand. This theory is against following rules or principles. Decisions and actions are taken on the basis of informed judgement in each particular instance within the context of each particular situation. Each context is unique regardless of how similar it appears to be to other situations, therefore each judgement will be unique. The duty of those taking the action is to be true to themselves. This theory is of little use to health workers as it advocates making arbitrary decisions. Also, in most cases health workers' professional responsibilities over-ride their personal moral commitments. For example, a staunchly Roman Catholic person has no right in his or her capacity as a health worker to deny another person contraception, although it is the case that in certain circumstances conscientious objection may be recognised (Beauchamp and Childress 1989).

In the context of health care, and the range of settings in which this takes place, it is generally thought that there is a need for rules and principles of conduct to guide professionals. This is because of the complexity both of the organisation and of the social relationships which are established within it (Seedhouse 1992). Rules and principles are seen to facilitate the need for rapid decision-making which at the same time adheres to the principle of justice.

Rule deontology

This states that an individual's decisions and actions should be based on a set of rules and that these should be followed without exception, regardless of outcomes. Following rules usually means that actions are predictable. The difficulty with this theory is that it offers little or no guidance on how to choose between rules which may be in conflict in a given situation. Although certain actions are right or wrong in themselves, their rightness or wrongness has to be weighed against the consequences.

Further variations on the deontological theme are as follows.

Acting in accord with nature

This perspective holds that some acts are natural and others are unnatural. Unnatural acts are wrong. There are many views as to which acts are unnatural. What is in accord with human nature is right, and what goes against human nature is wrong. This is only effective if we can identify human nature sufficiently precisely to say which actions are in accordance with human nature and which are not. Unfortunately it may not be possible to do this as many parts of human nature are at war with each other.

Doing God's will

This position argues that right actions are those which are in agreement with God's will and wrong actions are those which go against God's will. God's will as to how humans should behave is believed to be pre-ordained in several different ways. One view is that God's will is expressed in sacred books such as the Bible, and in proclamations such as the Ten Commandments. Acting rightly is following the rules, or learning how to apply the rules. God's will can also be revealed directly to individuals through their personal relationship with God. Another view is that God's will is revealed in examples of ideal behaviour such as the lives and actions of Christ and the saints. Finally, there is the belief that God's will is revealed in proclamations by church leaders, such as the Pope, through such means as papal encyclicals.

Given the different ways in which God's will is believed to be revealed, it is not surprising that people from different religious traditions disagree as to what God's will is and how it should be applied in particular circumstances. Agreement to act in accordance with God's will does not always produce agreement about what should be done in a given situation. What is a good reason for doing something according to one moral view may not be a good reason within another moral view. The fact that an action is believed to be in accordance with God's will does not give a non-believer a moral obligation to carry it out. However, a significant number of people believe that an act is right if it is based on God's law and wrong if it has been forbidden by God's law. This raises difficulties as people understand different things by 'God's law' and people have different perceptions of God depending on their religious beliefs. This also does not help people to decide which God-given law should be followed in which context.

Generalising from these different themes within deontology, it can be seen that certain acts and principles are considered to be moral in themselves. Such acts and principles ought to be carried out and adhered to by all human beings (Seedhouse 1992). The truly moral act is not influenced by social benefit or self-interest. It is held that all human beings are entitled to mutual respect. Although there are individual differences between people, we have a sufficient number of features in common to allow us to draw the conclusion that we are all in the same boat. From this it follows that we should not act towards another person differently from the way we like to be treated ourselves (Seedhouse 1992). Actions may be wrong in themselves either because they are actions that have certain qualities; or they are actions of a certain sort, such as deliberately taking life, or deliberate and unnecessary cruelty. On the other hand, honesty, truthfulness, fairness and justice make actions right in themselves. This is because actions based on these principles are viewed as positive duties. At the same time actions such as not telling lies, not keeping promises and so on are seen as negative duties. The intention behind these duties is to ensure that we avoid actions that are wrong in themselves. The notion of honesty and truthfulness, which is a firm principle of rule deontologists, means not deceiving people.

There is a further principle which is essential to the deontological perspective, that of justice and fairness. This can mean:

1 Regarding all people as equally valuable regardless of their age, race, gender, colour, sexual orientation, nationality, religious or political views. It is fair and just to consider the well-being of each person as equally important and so treat everyone alike.

2 Treating people impartially by applying rules or principles that are known and respected. For example, it would appear unfair or unjust to reprimand one individual for breaking a rule if others are not equally reprimanded, or if no one knew that the action was against the rules.

3 Treating people in the way they deserved, by giving them their just desserts or by rewarding them according to their merit. For example, it may be unfair and unjust to promote someone who is lazy over another who is conscientious. Viewing certain actions as right or wrong is done on an intuitive level. It is impossible to explain why these actions are right or wrong (Rowson 1990).

In general terms actions which indicate respect for people are morally right and actions that 'use' people are morally wrong. Moral motivation is concerned with performing the right actions and avoiding the wrong ones. Therefore morality is a matter of carrying out your duty to perform or avoid actions that are right or wrong in themselves. The motivation to act morally is the concern to perform actions because they are right and not for any other reason, in other words 'duty for duty's sake'. In this, morality is its own reward. According to this view, we are motivated by morality. We want to tell the truth because this is morally right in itself and therefore rewarding. However, the situation can arise where we do not tell the truth because it may lead to something else we value, such as being admired by friends. From the deontological perspective it can be seen that if the motivation for a person acting honestly is so that they will be admired, then they are not motivated by morality. In such a case they would only be valuing honesty or truthfulness because it happened to be useful, rather than acting morally as an end in itself. This would mean that the person was not acting morally.

Those who see 'respect for persons' as a foundation upon which all ideas of morality are built, claim that this can be used to explain why certain acts are right or wrong in themselves. Actions of honesty, fairness and justice are right because they show respect for the individual. Acts which are dishonest, unfair, unjust and cruel are wrong because they do not value or respect people. If someone lies to you that person is reducing your capacity to understand your surroundings. As this capacity is a valuable part of you as a person, they are failing to respect you as a person. Therefore they are manipulating or 'using' your intelligence for their own purposes.

The notions of right or wrong are fundamental to this view, as is duty and obligation.

The emphasis here is not upon the action but on the person. Moral rules or imperatives state that you should act only according to that maxim (conventional moral rule), by which you can at the same time will that it should become universal law. This means that every time people are about to make a moral decision they must first ask, 'What is the rule authorising this act?' Second they must ask, 'Can it become a universal rule for all human beings to follow?' This emphasises the freedom of the individual and the duty of the one for the many. A right action is only right if it is done out of a sense of duty, and the only good thing without any qualification is a person's goodwill, that is, the will to do what one knows to be right. The supreme principle of morality/practical imperative is to treat every rational being, including yourself, always as an end and never as a mere means (Tschudin 1992). This concept is drawn from Kant's proposition of the 'categorical imperative', which is the rule by which all rules must be tested.

ETHICAL PROBLEMS ASSOCIATED WITH BEHAVIOURAL TECHNIQUES

Karasu (1981) outlined the ethical problems of behaviour modification. The ethical issues revolve first around the behaviour therapist's view of the origins of human behaviour, and second in its alleged potential for contributing to a dehumanising or diminution of the individual. A third issue is behaviour modification's failure to view the person as a whole by separating people from their problems/symptoms, as this fosters a mechanistic and reductionist model of human beings. The therapist acts through manipulating the social environment with the aim of producing normalised behaviours. In this it is thought that behaviour modification has more profound ethical implications than other treatments as it does not expand the awareness of the individual receiving therapy. Other psychotherapies focus upon helping people to understand the meaning of their symptoms.

The principle merit of behaviour modification techniques resides in their efficient and impersonal application, without necessarily dealing with the troubling implications of what the person's behaviours might mean. Value judgements are limited to the extent to which a particular behaviour deviates from the norm. This contrasts with techniques where there is either an implicit or explicit valuation of the person's capacity to act morally. The method works relatively quickly so there is little time to contemplate the repercussions of the treatment. However, the degree to which behaviour can be altered without the intervening influence of the person's own cognitive valuation has been greatly exaggerated. It cannot succeed if the person does not wish to change.

Behavioural methods are particularly adept at meeting the needs of society over those of the individual. These methods may be used to increase conformity and reinforce social norms while reducing assertiveness and non-conforming behaviours, and at the same time defining deviant behaviour. Aversive conditioning and negative reinforcement raise major ethical difficulties such as the question of when the ends can justify the means.

DECISION-MAKING

Carers face many moral dilemmas created by conflicting moral principles that in turn generate conflicting demands. However, if the conflict exists between self-interest and a moral obligation then this is not a moral dilemma. Moral dilemmas only exist where two or more moral considerations will result in opposing or contradictory courses of action. For example, such a dilemma arises where the right of personal freedom conflicts with the right of others not to be injured. Decisions in such cases are justified by moral rules. These rules in turn are justified by principles which can be defended by ethical theory. However, conflicts and tensions may also arise between different carers when they are faced with making such decisions because individual beliefs are affecting the interpretation of the situation. Thus a difference in opinion about which course of action to take may arise not only from disagreement about the relevant moral code of action derived from ethical theories, but also from our own beliefs (Beauchamp and Childress 1989).

A decision is only ethical if it is based on something firm. The theories of ethics attempt to supply this firm base. The ethical question is 'what is the right thing to do?'. A decision therefore must take account of what is meant by 'right'. Each of the theories discussed above will provide an answer based upon different basic principles (Tschudin 1992).

Utilitarianism defines right in terms of the good produced by the

consequences of an action. The probable results of performing
results of performing various actions are calculated and the one
which maximises benefit over harm is chosen. Right, from this perspective, will conform to the greatest happiness principle. Actions
are right in proportion to their potential to promote happiness, and
wrong in proportion to their potential to produce the reverse of
happiness. In this sense happiness is equated with pleasure and the
absence of pain, while unhappiness is equated with pain and the
privation of happiness. As stated earlier the basic tenet of utilitarianism is to achieve the greatest good for the greatest number.
Thus all actions are future-oriented, and morality does not depend
on any historical duty. The difficulty with this view is how to decide
what is the good to be created, or what is pain and how to avoid it.
The British welfare system lies firmly within the utilitarian perspective (Tschudin 1992).

In contrast, the deontological perspective states that actions are
right in themselves and defines right by considering intrinsic
features of actions largely independent of consequences. A decision
therefore depends on the nature of the action itself. In addition,
this theory considers that the interests and human rights of a person
are of primary importance and that the purpose of right lies in
serving the cause of justice.

When making decisions therefore, the following notions are
important. People have their own minds and, based on their understanding of a situation, they can: think about what to do; weigh up
the pros and cons; reach conclusions as to what they think is worth-
while; form intentions and purposes; make decisions; carry out
decisions; and pursue objectives.

To aid decision-making using ethical theories one needs clear
principles which embody and cover the main tenets of the theories.
Such principles do not provide us with fixed answers. Rather, by
directing our thinking towards particular points for consideration,
they help towards the achievement of consensus over what ought to
be done in different circumstances. Thiroux (1980) has identified
five such principles. These principles, listed below, are inter-
dependent and are not hierarchical in nature.

(a) the value of life;
(b) goodness or rightness;
(c) justice or fairness;
(d) truth-telling or honesty;
(e) individual freedom.

The principle of value of life

Human beings should revere life and accept death. Most, if not all, systems of morality have an injunction against killing. This principle stands first because life is held both in common and uniquely by all human beings. Life is one thing people have in common but each person experiences it differently. The other four principles stand in relation to this basic one. This principle does not mean 'life at all costs' or that quantity comes before quality, indeed it is stated that people should accept death (Thiroux 1980). It is argued that people should neither be killed nor have their life preserved without their informed consent, unless there is very strong justification.

The principle of goodness or rightness

This principle logically comes before the other three as the question of good and right is the basis of ethics. Many ethical theories are built on the assumptions that everyone has, or should have, some idea or value of good. As society changes so its values change and consequently what it values as good. Good is not only abstract but relates to other people. This principle demands that we promote goodness over badness, that we cause no harm or badness and that we prevent badness or harm.

The principle of justice or fairness

It is stated that when actively doing good is not possible, then the principle of not doing harm should be maintained. In addition to this it is felt that we cannot be good without being just or fair. Good people should try to distribute the benefits from being good and doing right. Thus the most ethical, just and fair way to determine who receives what would be a fairly conducted lottery as this would not discriminate against anyone on the basis of mental ability, gender or so on. This egalitarian approach would appear to be the most just in distributing good and right. Egalitarianism is an important part of the principle of justice but is difficult to apply. Upholding the principle of justice means that we strive at least to do no harm.

The principle of truth-telling or honesty

Communication is the vehicle for ethics. The issue of truth-telling is fundamental to being ethical, for in order for communication to be sustained it has to be based on truthfulness. However, it takes two individuals to communicate the truth, one who speaks and one who listens and hears. Hearing is therefore crucial for truth-telling. How people perceive their truth may be more important than the truth they are told. Any act of deception or untruth is harmful to relationships. Truth is not simply a fact but incorporates the many perceptions around the fact which get built up over time.

The principle of individual freedom

The principle of freedom does not mean that we do as we please but provides the freedom to act morally (Thiroux 1980). We need to use freedom to preserve life, do right, be good, act justly and tell the truth. If we did not have the freedom to do this, or reject it, there would be no morality. Therefore, neither this principle, nor the other four, can stand alone. Each person is unique and will express the other four principles in his or her own way. This is in contrast to earlier theories where individual freedom had no clear place. Freedom is not a licence to do as we please, but freedom to act morally (Thiroux 1980).

CASE STUDY: JANE THOMAS AND MARK BLACK

Some forms of rule utilitarianism and rule deontology lead to virtually identical principles, rules and recommended actions. It is possible from both perspectives to defend the same principles such as respect for autonomy and justice, and rules such as truth-telling. It is also possible to assign these rules and principles the same weight in cases of conflict. However, the major difference is that utilitarians believe that the principle of utility justifies all other principles and rules, while deontologists believe some principles and rules are justified by reasons other than utility and are binding, even if they cannot be reliably predicted to maximise utility.

This similarity in recommended actions between the two main ethical theories may be due to the application of a different set of ethical principles which is more widely used in Britain (Gillon 1986) than that espoused by Thiroux. These four principles are:

(a) the principle of respect for autonomy;
(b) the principle of justice;
(c) the principle of beneficence;
(d) the principle of non-maleficence.

Tschudin notes that a further condition is usually added to these four principles; that is, respect for the person. While these principles differ little from those outlined by Thiroux, they do include the addition of the principle of non-maleficence (or the avoidance of doing harm). However, non-maleficence does not take priority over beneficence (or doing good). The scope of non-maleficence is general, encompassing all other people, whereas the scope of beneficence is more specific, applying only to some people (Tschudin 1992).

The objective of this section is to discuss these principles in the context of a case study which will be used to highlight particular concerns and tensions. In health care non-maleficence may be more applicable than beneficence. Medications and other treatments cause harm in the interest of improving health. If the only consideration were to be beneficence at all costs then these treatments would not be administered. Non-maleficence therefore is an important principle for practitioners (Gillon 1986). For example, it is possible to do harm by truth-telling as well as by lying.

Jane is a 24-year-old woman with a moderate degree of learning disability. She lives with her boyfriend Mark who is 22 years old and also has some learning disability. Mark works at a large supermarket, stocking shelves. He enjoys his work and gets on well with his work mates. Jane works at the local laundry. She also enjoys her job and has a few friends there. Jane has worked at the laundry for four years and is considered to be very reliable and to work hard. Jane and Mark have known each other for what seems to be all their life and have lived together for three years. They went to the same school and although Mark is younger they were in the same class. When Jane left school she went to the adult day service. She did not particularly like it there and spent most of her time doing leisure activities. This meant that she did not have anything special to do in her leisure time.

However, one of the staff at the day service took a particular interest in Jane and worked with her to help her get the job in the laundry. This job gave Jane a greater degree of independence and meant that she had her own money. It also meant that she now had something to do with her leisure time as she could no longer do leisure activities during her working hours. Mark was fortunate and when he left school he started work at the supermarket and so he did not attend the day service centre. Initially he worked part-time, but for the past two years he has worked full-time.

Jane and Mark enjoyed the same activities while at school and when Jane left school they continued to meet in the evenings and at weekends to participate in these activities. They enjoyed listening to music, dancing and swimming. Mr and Mrs Thomas, Jane's parents, and Mr and Mrs Black, Mark's parents, were quite happy for them to spend time with each other. However, when they realised that the couple wanted to live together, both sets of parents objected, despite the fact that both Jane and Mark were working and financially independent of their parents.

The parents tried to stop them seeing each other and would not let them meet at night. This upset Jane and Mark, but they tried to make sure that they had lunch at the same time. At least this meant that they could spend approximately fifteen minutes together. The time together was short as they had to meet half-way between their respective workplaces. Eventually they started meeting after work before going home, which meant that they arrived home later than usual. They usually got told off by their parents for this. This made both Jane and Mark angry, uncomfortable and humiliated, because they felt they were being treated like children.

It was at this time that Mark and Jane decided to apply to the local council for accommodation with the idea that they wished to set up home together. One of Jane's friends told her how to do this. Eventually they were allocated a two-bedroomed flat. It wasn't in a very nice area, but it was close to work and it meant that they could be together at last. They purchased the furniture and household goods, mostly from second-hand shops. They could not afford new furniture but what they purchased was clean and functional. They moved into the flat as soon as they could.

Approximately six months after they moved into the flat, Jane's parents decided to visit to see how she was. They were surprised to find that the flat was clean and tidy and that both Jane and Mark were healthy and happy. After this visit they kept in touch and enjoyed visiting the couple. Mark and Jane always knew that they were different from most people, because they went to a special school and they had visits from a social worker. They were not sure why the social worker visited, but they did not mind, as the visits were not frequent.

Mark and Jane decided that they would like to start a family, just one child as they didn't think they could cope with any more than this. They went to the library and borrowed books about having a baby. However, the books used long words and Jane and Mark could not really understand them. They decided to discuss the idea with the doctor at the family planning clinic Jane used, and so they went to see her. She advised them to discuss it with their own doctor and they did so. Their general practitioner was concerned that they would not be able to cope or to understand the physical changes that Jane would experience. In view of this he asked Jane and Mark if they would talk to the community nurse about their decision, and again they agreed.

The community nurse for people with a learning disability visited Jane and Mark and explained the things which they could not understand in the books. She also borrowed videos for them from the health authority, that showed a baby being born. This did not affect Jane and Mark's decision to have a baby and the community nurse told the doctor this. Jane and Mark asked the community nurse if all prospective parents had to talk to nurses and doctors and read books and watch videos, and if so why were there so many uncaring parents around. The nurse explained that not all people did receive this service but everyone involved wanted to make sure that Mark and Jane knew what they were doing.

Jane became pregnant and went to see the doctor, who confirmed the pregnancy and said he wanted to see them both. When Jane and Mark went to see the doctor he had a woman with him, who was introduced to them as Mrs Palmer, a social worker. The doctor spoke about something called 'a termination' and asked them if they wanted one. Jane did not know what this meant, but she understood that if they had it then they would not have the baby. She did not know why the doctor asked them this as he already knew that they wanted this baby; after all, they had told him this months ago. Jane didn't want to see the doctor again, but she was told that she had to so that they could make sure that the baby was all right. Jane found this confusing because the doctor did not want her to have the baby, otherwise he wouldn't have spoken about the termination.

Jane's parents were not happy about her being pregnant but Jane thought that they would change their minds as they had done about her and Mark living together. Mrs Palmer became a regular visitor and both Jane and Mark found this unsettling. They wished that she would go away. Mrs Palmer finally told them that the baby would probably be taken away from Jane after the birth. This upset Jane and Mark and they wanted to know why. When Mrs Palmer explained that they probably would not be able to care for the baby properly, Jane and Mark objected that they were not being given the chance and asked how Mrs Palmer knew they would not be able to cope.

Jane gave birth to a healthy baby girl and both she and Mark were over-joyed. Prior to the baby being discharged from hospital a case conference was held. This set out to consider Mark and Jane's circumstances and to decide whether they should keep their child. This posed a wide range of ethical issues.

It is useful to stop at this point and reconsider the decisions which have been made so far in the context of the principles suggested by Gillon. First, respect for autonomy would support the idea that the choices of indi-viduals, as long as they do not impinge on the freedom of others, should be promoted. Here Jane and Mark are making decisions about seeing each other and about the way they wish to see their relationship develop. They have also decided, after some thought, to have a child.

From a deontological perspective the rights of these two individuals to make this decision should be promoted. Others, such as the parents, would be seen to have a duty not to frustrate the decision so long as it was clear that it was a rational choice, freely made and entered into without coercion. If the parents sought to frustrate the decision because it caused them worry then they could be seen as acting immorally. On the other hand, the utilitarian perspective would take into account the concerns of the parents and the possibility that there would be general costs to society in the future. These costs would be related to an anticipation of the degree of support Jane and Mark might need in living together and caring for a child. In this case the principle of autonomy would probably lend support for Jane and Mark keeping their child.

With respect to the principle of justice, here again the question would be justice, or fairness, for whom? The deontological perspective would consider whether it was fair that this couple should be able to decide to live together and care for their child. In doing so the decision would focus upon duty, and would consider the couple's feelings for each other, their ability to respect each other and to share. It would also consider their duty towards their child and whether they would carry this duty out. This perspective may raise issues about marriage and the wider duty of the couple to the moral order of society.

The utilitarian perspective would consider different issues in the context of fairness. Being future-orientated it would question the fairness of the ongoing worry that Jane and Mark's parents may have about the relationship, and their ability to bring up their grandchild. It may also raise doubts about the capability of Jane and Mark to share and to support each other, especially when things are difficult. In such an eventuality it might argue that the responsibility for resolving a breakdown in their relationship would fall to others. Again, it is likely that in these circumstances the principle of justice would support Jane and Mark as they are the parents, and it would be 'natural' for them to bring up their child.

The principle of beneficence argues that we should act to do good. This of course is a major commitment of the utilitarian perspective where good is seen as maximising happiness. In this case it can be seen that for Jane and Mark happiness would be promoted through them living together and caring for their child, but that this might not promote happiness for their respective parents. There is also the anticipation of future happiness or good. In discussing beneficence from a utilitarian perspective, good has to be considered in terms both of its magnitude and of the numbers of people involved. Here it may be seen that while happiness is created through Jane and Mark continuing to care for their child, this may be out-weighed by the good achieved by not allowing this. That is, more good would be created for more people, such as the grand-parents and the service agencies, by not allowing Jane and Mark to care for their child.

From the deontological perspective there is a different focus on the idea of beneficence. Good in this case would not be related to happiness. Rather it would relate to whether or not the actions involved can be considered to be inherently right, as good can only be served by promoting right acts. The question here would be to decide what is right; whether Jane and Mark should be allowed to care for their child or prevented from doing so. Duty would usually hold that parents have the right to care for their child, as long as they prove to be competent, but the question then has to be: what good is served by them being prevented from doing this? As noted above, beneficence is concerned with the specific circumstances rather than more general concerns. Here duty can be considered in relation to Jane and Mark and to their baby, and the decision may concern our duty to each of them.

With respect to the principle of beneficence, therefore, Jane and Mark's position may be more difficult to support from both ethical perspectives. The concern over the baby's welfare would also enter the discussion. The future orientation of utilitarianism would require a cost-benefit analysis of the problems of removing the baby now against the possibility of having to remove it later. The significant bonding that would have taken place by then would make the situation much more traumatic for all concerned. In this case it may be felt that good is served by acting now rather than being forced to act later.

The fourth principle, that of non-maleficence, relates to more general concerns. Here it is seen that actions should avoid harm, and again the two perspectives would have different positions upon what constitutes harm. For utilitarianism, harm would be related to unhappiness, and the question would be whether our acts had the potential to produce a general unhappiness. In the case of Jane and Mark, non-maleficence would relate to whether a general unhappiness would be caused by them caring for their child. For example, they may not be able to cope, causing a general anxiety about what to do. Or their parents might resort to the legal process to prevent them caring for their child, possibly through some form of custody application. This might have an unsettling effect with consequences for the relationships between the couple and those who might become involved in their lives. There might be other consequences, for example problems in Mark's workplace, the expense of the legal process, press coverage, and the possibility that Jane and Mark's specific case gets lost in some wider, and for them, impersonal debate about rightᶜ

From the deontological perspective the issue of non-maleficence would be related to the idea of duty. Here the decision as to whether Jane and Mark should live together and care for their child might raise questions over the extent to which it could be universally applied. Will the decision create a precedent which cannot be met in all cases? Or might it create a confusion about where duty lies?

Again, as with the principle of beneficence, both perspectives raise difficult issues. The future orientation of utilitarianism would hold that the greater general harm might occur by not acting now. The confusion over duty, that is, whether this is towards Jane and Mark or towards the baby, would tend to give prominence to the utilitarian position.

The final principle for consideration is respect for the person. This, in many ways, raises questions over the process of reaching a decision over the form of action appropriate where there is a moral dilemma. That is, is it undertaken in a way that maintains the dignity of the person? In the case of Mark and Jane this would relate to issues such as the extent to which they participated in the decision-making process. It would focus upon whether all possible courses of action were given a fair and unbiased hearing. It would involve the feelings and aspirations of Mark and Jane, and whether they were told the truth about what was going on. It would also consider the manner in which the process was conducted, for example were they treated as children, or referred to in devaluing terms.

CONCLUSION AND SUMMARY

It is time to return to the case study to consider the decision finally taken. This was that in the interests of the baby she should be placed in a foster home prior to adoption. Jane and Mark were devastated and Jane needed treatment for depression. They did not see their daughter again. Instead they were left to rebuild their lives and face a future without the child they loved and wanted.

The ethical dilemma described in the case study is one which emphasises the difficult nature of judgements made within health and other caring services. This chapter has proposed that in order to facilitate the decision-making process it is necessary to utilise ethical theories, but these can result in different decisions. In this case the decision to remove the child can be seen to rest in the tensions between ideas of duty and happiness in two common ethical perspectives. These arise from the different interpretations the perspectives provide of the principles of beneficence and non-maleficence. Thus a utilitarian ethical decision was made, based upon a cost-benefit analysis and a prediction of the likely consequences of the action. However, from a deontological perspective, it could be argued that allowing a child to live with its natural parents is an intrinsically right action and therefore any decision to remove the child is morally wrong.

From the case study it can be seen that, while a knowledge of ethical theories might aid decision-making, this does not resolve the dilemma in itself. Rather, it can provide a basis upon which judgements can be made and against which such judgements can be explained and justified.

In conclusion, deontology is concerned with what the person ought to do, and the notion of obligation towards right and wrong conduct. The deontological perspective states that some actions are right or wrong in themselves. That is, there is something inherent in the action which makes it ethically right or wrong, reflected in such edicts as 'you should not commit murder'. On the other hand, the utilitarian perspective focuses upon consequences. These consequences should bring about the greatest good for the greatest number of people. As a result, some people may be disadvantaged, but this would be ethically acceptable as these people would be in the minority. Here the principle of the greatest good for the greatest number would be upheld.

Health, and care services generally, predominantly operate upon utilitarian ethical principles. Utilitarians argue that the principles of beneficence and non-maleficence provide the axis upon which morality can be based. This takes account only of what can be seen from an objective viewpoint, whereas morality is essentially personal and needs to include the participants' attitudes (Brown *et al.* 1992). While both utilitarian and deontological perspectives incorporate basic principles, these should be viewed only as guides to conduct at the general level, that is, reasons for acting or not acting in certain ways. Gillon (1986) offers a framework that allows for decision-making between the different guiding principles offered by the different ethical perspectives. However, it has to be noted that a principle will carry weight and shape people's decisions only if they believe in it.

KEY POINTS

Beneficence	Honesty
Consequentialism	Human Rights
Cost-benefit analysis	Justice
Decision-making	Morality
Deontology	Non-maleficence
Dilemmas	Rights
Duties	Truthfulness
Fairness	Utilitarianism

REFERENCES

Beauchamp, T. and Childress, J. (1989) *Principles of Biomedical Ethics*, 3rd edn, Oxford: Oxford University Press.

Block, S. and Chadaff, P. (1981) *Psychiatric Ethics*, Oxford: Oxford University Press.

Brown, J., Kitson, A. and Mcknight, T. (1992) *Challenges in Caring*, London: Chapman Hall.

Department of Health (DoH) (1990) *The N.H.S. and Community Care Act 1990*, London: HMSO.

Gillon, R. (1986) *Philosophical Medical Ethics*, Chichester: Wiley.

Hare, R. (1991) *Moral Thinking: Its Levels, Method and Point*, 2nd edn, Oxford: Clarendon Press.

Karasu, T. (1981) 'Ethical aspects of psychotherapy' in S. Block and P. Chadaff (eds), *Psychiatric Ethics*, Oxford: Oxford University Press.

Osmanczyk, E. (1985) *Encyclopedia of the United Nations*, London: Taylor and Francis.

Rowson, R. (1990) *An Introduction to Ethics for Nurses*, London: Scutari Press.

Seedhouse, D. (1992) *Ethics: the Heart of Health Care*, Chichester: Wiley.

Thiroux, J. (1980) *Ethics, Theory and Practice*, 2nd edn, Encino, California: Glencoe.

Tschudin, V. (1992) *Ethics in Nursing. The Caring Relationship*, London: Butterworth Heinemann.

FURTHER READING

Aroshar, M. (1980) 'Anatomy of an ethical dilemma: the theory, the practice', *American Journal of Nursing* 80(4): 653–63.

Beauchamp, T. and McCullough, L. (1984) *Medical Ethics, The Moral Responsibility of Physicians*, London: Prentice Hall.

Campbell, A. (1984) *Moral Dilemmas in Medicine*, Edinburgh: Churchill Livingstone.

Candee, D. and Puka, B. (1984) 'An analytical approach to resolving problems in medical ethics', *Journal of Medical Ethics* 10: 61–70.

Harris, J. (1987) 'Qualifying the value of life', *Journal of Medical Ethics* 13(3): 117–23.

Kleining, J. (1982) *Ethical Issues in Psychosurgery*, London: George Allen and Unwin.

Mill, J.S. (1967) *Utilitarianism*, London: Longman.

Smart, J. and Williams, B. (1973) *Utilitarianism: For and Against*, Cambridge: Cambridge University Press.

Chapter 4

Informed choice: from theory to practice

Tony Dix and Tony Gilbert

INTRODUCTION

This chapter discusses the concept of informed choice and the dilemmas it presents for health professionals involved in the lives of people with learning disabilities. It is important to establish the context within which the discussion takes place for, like many concepts, informed choice is multi-faceted and has legal, moral, ethical, as well as practical aspects. Much of the literature on the subject mainly concerns the requirement placed upon practitioners to obtain informed consent. The proposition here is that for any practitioner working with people with a learning disability there is an additional requirement. This is to ensure that all possible efforts are made to enable the people concerned to make an informed choice. For it is upon this basis only that informed consent can be achieved. The practitioner who intervenes without consent does so in a way that violates the principle of self-determination, and in so doing undermines the dignity of the person concerned. This is as true for individual interventions as it is for the development of total packages such as care management. But the concept of informed choice is problematic. What in fact constitutes an informed choice? How do we determine the costs and benefits of a particular choice? And, what do we do when apparent choices become disabling? These are all difficult and complex issues which need to be identified as being integral to the practitioner's role.

This discussion, while drawing on both legal and philosophical ideas, is concerned with the implications of informed choice for practice, and for the people who are subject to that practice. It should be noted that some of the terminology used in particular quotations is not that which is normally considered appropriate for contemporary services and that some quotations refer to particular types of practitioners. However, this is because of the need to maintain accuracy in quotation. In such cases, unless otherwise specified, the reader should take it that the subject is practitioners in general.

In exploring the concept of informed choice, this chapter will focus upon the process through which it is achieved, and the importance of education to this process (Fiesta 1991). It will also identify the critical importance of context (White 1989). This is not to deny the importance of informed choice as an outcome. Rather, it is an acknowledgement that in the context of services which are long-term, which involve complex aspects of human experience, and where the people involved may go through many changes while in contact with those services, there is a continuous need to re-affirm both informed choice and informed consent.

This chapter does not aim to provide either an ideal model for informed choice, nor to provide any other form of right answer. Instead, the intention is to unpack the complexity of the concept, and to consider ways of dealing in everyday circumstances with the requirement of competence associated with it. This locates informed choice as integral to the complex sets of inter-personal relationships which are achieved in human services.

It is also important to be clear that while the discussion will draw upon comment from legal practitioners it in no way sets out to be, nor should it be considered as, an informed legal opinion on the issue of informed choice. Rather, the chapter draws upon legal opinions from both Britain and the United States in an attempt to develop from them principles for practice. It is important for any-one who is involved with people with learning disabilities and who wishes to establish a legal opinion of the concept of informed choice, to seek this from qualified legal counsel. Likewise, this discussion is not a philosophical investigation.

Returning to the practical implications of informed choice, the discussion is based on the following structure. The first section of the chapter considers the emergence of informed choice as a doctrine that is considered, by some, to be the antithesis of paternalism. This is followed by an attempt to locate informed choice within a particular philosophical framework which sets up the notion of the rights and obligations of the responsible moral person. Once this philosophical base has been established, the chapter goes on to identify the constituent elements of informed choice through the use of a fictitious case study. This section is then developed by considering the possible safeguards and constraints resulting from the 'requirements' to demonstrate that information has been given, competence assessed, and the absence of coercion assured (White 1989). The final section considers the idea of risk. It identifies risk as an essential part of human experience promoting both dignity and growth and discusses how risk might be successfully managed.

THE EMERGENCE OF INFORMED CHOICE

In recent times the concept of informed choice has become important to people with learning disabilities who, through organisations such as People First and the growing advocacy movement (Crawley 1988), have articulated a call for more say in the way their lives develop. This mirrors a general reaction against paternalism in the practices of both social services (Croft and Beresford 1990) and medicine (Smith 1990).

Informed choice has also become a concern of professional practitioners and the wide range of other people involved in supporting people with learning disabilities. In many cases this represents a genuine attempt to include informed choice as a central principle of practice with individuals. However, it is also true that informed choice has become a condition of decisions made by people with learning disabilities to the extent that it can constrain their growth. An example of this might be where a decision made by a person with a learning disability is over-ruled by a professional, or other person, on the basis that the choice is uninformed. Coy argues: 'Health care professionals often conclude that the patient has made the "wrong" choice and that they, the professionals, are justified in overriding that choice' (Coy 1989: 829). It may of course be true that the particular choice involved could be harmful or life-threatening to the person concerned. Such examples provide the everyday tensions that exist between theory and practice in complex human services, and in the more complex environment of human interaction. However, the principle of normalisation, which has been adopted by many services and agencies working with people with learning disabilities, upholds the idea of choice as central to the accomplishments of that service:

Choice is the experience of autonomy both in small, everyday matters (e.g., what to eat or what to wear) and in large, life-defining matters (e.g., with whom to live or what work to do). Personal choice defines and expresses individual identity. Without focused effort to increase available options and provide support for decision making, people with severe handicaps will be passive and without voice or the ability to escape undesirable situations. People with severe handicaps can challenge others' ability to detect personal preferences; some may depend upon a guardian to choose their interests. Valued activities will increase the variety and significance of the choices that a person makes.

(O'Brien 1987: 177–8)

There is a further tension which arises in the emergence of the concept of informed choice. Multi-disciplinary care working, especially that with a health-care element, involves a wide range of practitioners. Here the tension lies in the nature of the resonsibilities of the medical practitioners who are members of the team. Such practitioners have a legal duty to demonstrate that informed choice has been achieved with respect to informed consent for a specific intervention. In this they may involve other practitioners, who also have legal and professional commitments to the principle of informed choice, to establish whether informed consent is in fact based upon an informed choice.

The tension arises from the fact that while these other practitioners have a duty to bring issues of informed choice to the notice of the medical practitioner concerned, in doing so they have to take care not to interfere with the process of informed consent with respect to the medical intervention. Hollowell and Eldridge state, in the context of nursing practice, that 'As a cautionary matter, however, a nurse's involvement in the consent process must not interfere with the physician–patient relationship' (Hollowell and Eldridge 1989: 29). Therefore it is important in human services for the practitioner to be clear over the nature and the source of a particular referral (Scott 1991).

In highlighting this latter point, the link between the emergence of informed choice and the medical profession needs to be identified. It is important not only because of the issues relating to multidisciplinary working, but also because it reflects the developing social reaction to paternalism in welfare services referred to above. This, it is argued, arises as a consequence of the role of medical practitioners as gatekeepers to these services, despite the fact that in many instances medicine holds no cure (Oliver 1990). It is probably because of this gatekeeping role that legal challenges based upon informed choice and informed consent have tended to concern the medical profession.

The history of informed choice is tied to that of informed consent which, as a practical concern, originates in the courts of the United States. These sought to establish the responsibilities of the physician. Smith (1990) identifies a case in the Californian courts in 1914 as one of the earliest examples. Here the following rule was established:

> a physician violates his duty to his patient and subjects himself to liability if he withholds any facts which are necessary to form the basis of an intelligent consent by the patient to the proposed treatment. . . . In discussing the element of risk a certain amount of discretion must be employed consistent with the full disclosure of facts necessary to an informed consent.
>
> (Smith 1990: 72)

A later opinion from Britain is provided by Marsh's discussion of informed consent. In a reference to Lord Scarman, he argues that,

> Scarman put it succinctly when he stated 'if a patient is fit to receive information and wishes to receive it, the doctor must "brief" the patient so that he can make a free and informed choice'. He went on to state that 'medical paternalism' is no longer acceptable as a matter of English law and that the 'sovereignty of the patient' was reinstated.
>
> (Marsh 1990: 603)

This particular quote is important as it clearly identifies that the concept of informed choice is integral to that of informed consent. It establishes that one is in fact the basis for the other.

It may be useful to consider this in the following terms. Professionals, or any other people or group of people, require the informed consent of any particular individual before they can intervene in any way in that person's life. In order for the individual to provide that consent they must have the time and information upon which to make an informed choice. This will determine whether they wish to accept or refuse that intervention, or in fact to choose another intervention which they feel is more suited to them.

This shift from paternalism to self-determination is viewed as representing a fundamental movement in the philosophy of care. It represents a move from a position where the professional is allowed to determine the amount of information, and the nature of that information, to a position which recognises self-determination.

This movement is often referred to as 'the professional standard' (paternalism) versus 'the patient standard' (self-determination). The philosophical issue is the subject of the following section of this chapter, while the issue of 'professional standard versus patient standard' will be discussed in the section on the practice of informed choice.

THE PHILOSOPHICAL BASE OF INFORMED CHOICE

Informed consent is a concept derived from a moral theory which upholds the 'principle of self-determination', alternatively referred to as the 'principle of autonomy', and it is upon this principle that it challenges the basis of paternalism. This moral theory, which Haber (1985) traces to Kant, provides that 'to respect an autonomous person is to take seriously [that] person's considered value judgements' (Haber 1985: 44). This applies regardless of whether you happen to agree or disagree with that person's judgement. In locating informed consent with Kant the concept is set within the traditions of firstly liberal, and later analytical, philosophy. These traditions have a long history of influence in Western society.

Central to the liberal tradition is the concept of 'personhood' which relates to the development of a rational being who, through the use of intellectual and social skills, demonstrates the capacity for 'reasonableness' (Patterson 1978). Reasonable people are therefore those who, first, are capable of acting morally through the making of choices, and second, have a 'life plan' through which they demonstrate their purpose in life and through which they achieve growth. To act morally a person must have the capacity to interpret situations and the behaviour of others in the context of a particular set of principles. The moral person then chooses between particular courses of action in a way that promotes these principles.

A person who acts expediently, or who merely follows rules, or who fails to act in the face of a moral imperative, is failing to act morally. The general principle is that persons should be seen as ends in themselves and not as the means to such ends. This can also be interpreted as 'do unto others as you would have done unto you'. In turn this sets up the deontological concept of duty which requires the practitioner to act in accordance with this principle.

Moreover, this duty falls upon the practitioner and the recipient in that they have obligations both to themselves and each other, and to the wider society. It is here that the relationship between rights and responsibilities can be seen to be established. In situations where a person is in some way incapacitated, and because of this is not able to demonstrate reasonableness, then that person is not a moral person. However, such individuals are moral subjects and as such have the right to be treated in accordance with the general principle.

The argument here is that to treat a person in a paternalistic way is to violate this general principle and therefore to act immorally, whether or not the person is incapacitated. This is a point made by Coy who argues:

> This duty means that a person should respect another person's decisions and not override those decisions, unless such decisions interfere with the rights of others. It means that no person should ever use another person as merely a means to achieve some result, even if that result will benefit the other person. When health care professionals act paternalistically, the patient is used as a means to achieve an end (ie, a good medical outcome) by overriding the patient's decisions, rather than respecting the patient as an individual with dignity.
>
> (Coy 1989: 829)

Smith (1990) considers that a further consequence of this rejection of paternalism is the move away from the use of terminology such as 'patient' to 'client' which, rather than being a purely semantic exercise, focuses upon the autonomy of the person.

This idea of the reasonable person who is capable of making rational choices forms the basis for the 'principle of self-determination' as a morally desirable state. It also sets up the requirement of 'competence' in relation to the concept of informed choice, an issue of practical concern that will be considered more fully later. The discussion will now move to consider the philosophical concept of the 'principle of beneficence' which, while it is often used in conjunction with the 'principle of autonomy', also provides the basis for the denial of informed consent and therefore the denial of informed choice. The 'principle of beneficence' upholds that:

> Because we care about the well-being of individual persons, we . . . grant a prominent place in the structure of our moral outlook to . . . the Principle of Beneficence. That principle, simply stated, holds that one ought to do good. Doing good means benefiting people, helping them, acting − out of respect for their interests − in a way that serves their interests.
>
> (Gorovitz 1982: 37)

The tension between beneficence and informed choice emerges due to the former's focus upon the need to produce the most favourable outcomes for the person. For it is not seen as essential to secure informed consent in cases where the particular intervention does not carry with it the potential for harm. In such cases the principle of the optimum good takes precedence (Coy 1989).

The caveat to this position is that if the most beneficial course has the possibility of harmful effects, then informed consent will be sought. Moreover, Coy argues that a moral dilemma arises when the practitioner is faced with a situation where a person's informed choice leads that person to select a behaviour which in the mind of the practitioner fails to meet the 'principle of beneficence'. This leads to a situation in which 'One alternative many health care providers choose is to override the patient's autonomous decision' (Coy 1989: 828). The result is that we return to paternalism.

To summarise the above section, it can be seen that both the dominant philosophical principles in the care environment have the potential to frustrate the exercise of informed choice by people with a learning disability. In respect to the 'principle of autonomy' the idea of competence can place the person with a learning disability in one of two positions. First, they may not be considered competent to make a choice, or second, they may have to demonstrate that their choice is informed before they can gain any assistance in exercising that choice. On the other hand the 'principle of beneficence' would allow for choices to be over-ridden where a professional felt that their choice failed to maximise the potential benefits. In either case there is a strong possibility that informed choice will be frustrated.

THE PRACTICE OF INFORMED CHOICE

The aim of this next section is to move on from the philosophical debate to begin to consider the implications for practice. This is done by identifying the constituent elements of informed choice. The connection between informed choice and informed consent continues to be emphasised; indeed, as stated earlier, the former is integral to the latter. The next section therefore opens with a discussion of the legal requirements for informed consent and the process through which it is secured.

However, before proceeding, it should be noted that the process through which informed choice is developed also has particular requirements and conditions. These relate to the nature of the information provided, the competence of the person, and to whether the choice was achieved without coercion (White 1989). These aspects of informed choice are addressed later in the chapter along with issues of documentation and the management of risk.

The elements of informed choice

In seeking to identify the elements of informed choice it is useful for clarity to focus briefly upon the legal aspects of the question. For while it is accepted that most of the legal decisions have been reached in the process of litigation concerning battery or negligence in respect of medical interventions, they do provide a guide for the more complex and inter-personal world of practice within community settings. Scott (1991), in discussing informed consent, argues that the legal position typically places the following requirements upon health care workers:

> To meet the legal requirements of informed consent, the following information typically must be disclosed to the patient before treatment, and all of the patient's questions must be answered.
>
> 1 Diagnosis or evaluative findings.
> 2 Nature of the recommended treatment.
> 3 Material (i.e., important to a patient's decision on treatment), or foreseeable risks or complications of the proposed treatment.
> 4 Prognosis if the treatment is carried out.
> 5 Reasonable alternatives to the proposed treatment, and attendant risks and prognosis if an alternative treatment is carried out.
> 6 Risks of foregoing treatment altogether.
>
> (Scott 1991: 12)

These elements of informed choice identified here relate to clinical interventions. Nevertheless, they are relevant to a number of different areas of practice involving people with learning disabilities and also identify a number of opportunities for the person both to make choices and, most importantly, to say no (Thorpe 1989).

However, it should be noted that in practice these elements of informed choice leading to informed consent, or non-consent, may not be mutually exclusive parts of the process. Indeed, the complex nature of human services implies that the relationship between the elements may be far from the linear progression proposed by Scott. In fact, the process may more closely resemble a spiral, with elements being revisited time and time again as the person grows. Also, in the context of human services, 'diagnosis or evaluative findings' are most likely to be the end-product in the assessment process occurring after the later stages identified by Scott. This is a crucial point in considering the length of time some people with learning disabilities may be associated with particular practitioners.

The next section discusses the elements of informed choice in the context of practice. This is done in two ways: first, each element is interpreted in a way appropriate to circumstances relating to the care of people with learning disabilities; second, each element is discussed with respect to a fictitious person, 'George Miles'.

George is a middle-aged man with a quite severe learning disability who lives in a small hospital which is situated in the middle of a rural town. George has lived here for over thirty years. However, while George has many friends in the hospital, he also has some friends who live in various parts of the town. Most of these people do not have a learning disability, some are members of his family but others are just people he has got to know over the years.

In his leisure time George likes to go to the shops, which he is able to do without assistance, or sometimes he chooses to visit his brother who also lives nearby. Occasionally he visits a friend on the other side of town and in this case a taxi has to be arranged to take him there. The issue is that George, who has often talked about moving out of the hospital into his own home, now has that opportunity. This has come about due to the planned closure of the hospital.

The proposal is that George move to three-bedroomed house on an estate in a village just outside the town. He will share the house with two other people who are also moving out of the hospital. One of these people George would describe as a friend, but the other is someone he finds a little difficult to get on with at times. The situation is that the hospital will be closed in three years time so there is no immediate pressure for George to accept this opportunity.

Diagnosis or evaluative findings

This element most closely relates to the assessment of needs and, in the context of working with people with learning disabilities, can often be clearly stated following a process which also secures the other elements required to demonstrate informed consent. This is an important issue for, in all cases, any credible evaluation has to involve the person concerned. This will often require that the care worker develop a deliberate strategy aimed at producing this evaluation.

In this case it can be seen that George has both expressed a wish to move to his own home and the developing circumstances will, in a fairly short period of time, make this a necesity. However, George has little experience of living in a small family-type home, other than that which he has obtained from visiting friends and family. And, of course, there has been the occasional stopover at his brother's house. This lack of experience itself need not be a barrier to assuring informed choice as it is often the case that people choose to do things they have no direct experience of.

As a note of caution, care workers who limit options to those the person has direct experience of will most probably further disable that person. In this sense the imagination of the person has a central role in informed choice. The challenge for the care worker is in drawing upon the concrete experiences, as well as the wishes, desires and imagination of the person concerned when seeking to empower that person to make an evaluation.

In ensuring informed choice as an outcome implicit within the evaluation or assessment, the care worker will need to draw upon a wide range of evidence. This may include discussions with George and any family and friends he wishes to be involved. The purpose is to build a picture of the kinds of things that are important to him. This process demands a partnership. With regard to care workers this relates to a particular form of relationship based upon trust and communication. Marsh describes this type of relationship as follows:

> Under the concept of fiduciary relationship, a person in whom another person has placed a special trust or confidence (as a result of his or her special training or expertise) is required to act in good faith and in the interests of the person reposing the trust or confidence.
>
> (Marsh 1990: 603)

The importance of this idea of fiduciary relationship is that it clearly identifies the partnership between the person and the care worker as one where there are special responsibilities, and obligations, of the care worker to the person. It acknowledges that before any personal relationship, friendship or emotional bond is established between these people, it is accepted that the care worker must act in the interests of the person. However this obligation is only reciprocated via the general principle. So while it is quite probable

that the 'evaluative findings' or 'assessment of need' will support
the idea of George's move, the obligation requires that informed
choice has to have been secured. In this it is essential that the
following elements are fully tested.

The nature of the recommended treatment

This element points to the necessity for the person to have gained a
thorough appreciation of the effects of a particular set of evaluative findings upon the life-style of the person concerned. This
demands that the care worker make a careful analysis of the likely
course of a particular intervention. In this case the care worker
would have to identify all of the knock-on effects of the proposed
move. The fact that George has been living in one place for a long
time will hold a number of challenges both for him and the care
worker. From the brief description it can be seen that George's
experiences are of a very particular kind, and he has little
experience of living in situations similar to those proposed. However, it should be possible to develop specific experiences for
George in order for him to gain an appreciation of what will
happen.

These experiences may include spending some time with the other
two people, possibly on a holiday, to see if they get along. This
would also involve discussion and reflection between the care
worker and George with regard to what it might be like to have to
make daily or weekly choices over household arrangements, and
ideas such as having to agree certain choices with the others.
George may also have concerns regarding living with just two other
people. He may want to know where there is help or assistance if
he, or one of the other people, should need it. He may want to
know what he could do if they fall out, and that falling out is something that happens.

Other possible experiences would relate to the physical and social
environment of the proposed new home. Here George may wish to
visit the village to familiarise himself with the local area. Further
experiences that might prove valuable are things such as travelling
on public transport between the village and the town, spending
some time in the local pub, and looking at the types of local activity
that George might wish to join in. George may also wish to take
some of his family or friends to the village to show them where he
will live and to assure himself that they will continue their contact.

These are all fairly concrete experiences but there is also a need to consider more subjective aspects such as George's wishes and aspirations.

In this the care worker could develop discussions with George about issues such as his personal belongings and the things that are important to him in his present environment, such as photographs, possibly a pet, the garden, a quiet spot on a bench. Other issues might relate to the possibilities of personal space and how much of this personal space he will have if he chooses to move. Issues of privacy and personal relationships are also important, as are the possibilities that such a move may have in terms of new opportunities.

Material or foreseeable risks

This element can be seen as raising the issue of the possible costs to the person, and it should be noted that this might relate to emotional, psychological, physical, social or financial costs. Here the care worker has a particular responsibility, for one of the key tests in the concept of informed consent is that of the 'materiality of risk standard' (Smith 1990). This is also known as the 'reasonable person' test, or the 'reasonable patient' test. This test sets the scope of the practitioner's duty as being determined by the client's right to decide, rather than professional custom. In a legal sense this 'Holds that, for a plaintiff to prevail, it must be shown that a reasonable person in his or her position would not have consented to the procedure if properly informed' (Cushing 1991: 18). This test has increasingly replaced the older test known as the 'professional standard' in which the duty is upon the practitioners to decide what information they will disclose. The 'professional standard' states that a practitioner must disclose to the client that information which another practitioner in similar circumstances would have disclosed.

In the context of George's move such a condition may be said to have arisen if, for example, George moved to the house only to find that the area opposite the house was a place where a gang of unemployed youths regularly hang out, it being well-known that George had a fear of gangs and noisiness, even if they are quite harmless. The consequence of this situation could be that George refused to go out and became very depressed. If it could be shown, first, that had the care worker researched the area properly then it would have been established that the site had been a regular meeting place for many years, and second, that if George had known this he would not have moved, then it is likely that the practitioner would fail the 'reasonable person' test.

Another important consideration here is what might be seen as complications. Again these would have to stand the 'reasonable person' test. In the case of George's move, suppose it was found that the situation of his new area meant that he had to rely upon public and other forms of transport rather than walking. This, in turn, might result in George becoming very over-weight and increasingly less mobile, with the consequence that he became almost house-bound. It might well be asked if this consequence could have been foreseen. If the answer is yes, and if it was likely that George, had he been informed that in a period of months he would no longer be able to get about, would have then decided against the move, it might be argued that the care worker had failed in the duty to promote an informed choice.

From the consideration of this element it is clear that practitioners have to be very thorough in their assessment of the potential costs to the person of a particular intervention. In cases where there are potential costs these need to be clearly identified and care taken that the person makes the decision in the clear knowledge of these potential costs. In certain circumstances where the potential benefits out-weigh the risks a strategy is designed to manage the risk. This issue of risk-taking and risk management will be discussed later in this section and also in the final section on dilemmas in choice.

Prognosis if the treatment is carried out

This element relates to the benefits the person is most likely to gain by choosing a particular intervention. This has to take account of the period of time it might take for such benefits to mature. These benefits have also to be weighed against the potential costs identified in the discussion above. This idea of prognosis is especially difficult when dealing with the complex inter-related aspects of a person's life chances. These are subject to change as a consequence of the person's growth, with needs and ambitions changing over time.

The consequences of radical changes such as George's move to another home could bring opportunities in a couple of years' time that cannot be foreseen today. People are also subject to the changes brought about by the decisions of others; for example, personal relationships form and break, friends make choices that move them away, care workers come and go. Then there are the wider changes related to society. The closure of the hospital where George lives is an example. At the present time patterns of employment and patterns of services are continuing to change.

Therefore in the context of prognosis, George's move is difficult to assess. There is also the question of the criteria against which this assessment is made. Here O'Brien's (1987) framework of 'service accomplishments', referred to earlier (page 90), has provided a popular tool through which this type of question is organised. This framework is often supplemented by a further set of categories, relating to residence, leisure and occupation, in order to construct a matrix which then poses questions about discrete areas of a person's life.

However, there is a need to provide a note of caution. This type of framework is designed to evaluate services. Therefore there is a danger that the 'general principle', referred to earlier, which establishes the philosophical base of informed choice, could be undermined. This 'general principle' states that people should be viewed as ends in themselves and not the means to an end. In focusing upon services there is a danger that people do become only the means to an end. Chappell (1992), writing from a sociological perspective, makes the following point:

> Quality studies have concentrated upon issues that are important to professionals: notably, how staff can utilise normalisation to construct quality of care or quality of life in residential settings, often for people leaving long-stay institutions. Furthermore, the definitions of quality of care and quality of life for people with learning difficulties have been dominated by the normalisation principle rather than the views of service users.

> (Chappell 1992: 40)

As can be seen from the discussion, the idea of prognosis is problematic. However, this does not mean that practitioners cannot work with the person with learning disability to establish the most likely set of outcomes. Care needs to be taken that these outcomes are realistic and that they are set within meaningful time frames. It also returns the discussion to the concept of process, in that people are likely to need ongoing support in order to adjust their lives to changes and to take advantage of previously unseen opportunities. For George this means that he will need the ongoing support of a care worker with whom the fiduciary relationship has been established.

Reasonable alternatives

This element relates to the possibility that there are likely to be other interventions that have the potential of achieving either a similar outcome through a different course of action, or a different outcome that will also meet the need. And, as noted previously, the complexity of human services makes the likelihood of alternatives very strong. Practitioners need to consider carefully the possible alternatives, especially in the context of working with people with learning disability, as they will need to be as thorough in respect of these options as in the case of the preferred option. However, the demands of time and the need to provide a serious consideration of the alternatives means that some options will most probably be discarded sooner than other options.

In George's case there may be other options that do not involve him moving out of town. However, these may involve him living with a larger group of people, or in an area he does not like very much. Alternatively there may be an option that requires him to move some miles away. Some of these moves might be happening soon, while others may be some time in the future.

Risks of forgoing treatment altogether

This element relates to the implications for the person of not making a choice. In some cases this might provide a real and meaningful strategy for the person. This has led to the emergence of the principle that Henry (1990) describes as the 'doctrine of informed refusal'. She argues that:

> Over the last decade, the legal principle of the doctrine of informed refusal has emerged from lawsuits seeking to recover damages arising from the failure of a health care provider (including the nurse practitioner) to inform the patient of the harmful consequences of not performing a test or procedure.
>
> (Henry 1990: 66)

This idea of the doctrine of informed refusal again highlights the obligations inherent within the fiduciary relationship. The onus is upon the practitioner to ensure that not only is the person's choice an informed one with respect to the alternative on offer, but also that the person is informed in the context of not making a choice. This means that care workers have to assure themselves that the person is not declining an option because of a fear of the unknown, or because more time is needed, or the particular options are fairly meaningless to the person because of previous experiences. The person may also have some unfounded fears regarding the consequences of accepting a particular option. Again, it can be seen that the test of the 'reasonable person' applies.

One of the most difficult types of situation that arises in the context of informed refusal is that where a person declines opportunities for growth, or adopts strategies that inhibit growth. For example, individuals might decline any opportunities which cause them to get out of bed, or they may decide to stop washing and changing their clothes. In both cases opportunities for growth are likely to be inhibited. The dilemma for the practitioner is whether these choices or refusals meet the criteria of being informed. For, if they do not, then the principle of 'self-determination' cannot be argued as being promoted. However, the judgement that a refusal is not informed does not provide the practitioner with the justification to use coercion. Rather it sets the obligation of the fiduciary relationship as being one where the practitioner must strengthen his or her efforts to promote informed choice.

In George's case he may be reluctant to move because the hospital has been his home for many years and represents all that is familiar. Moreover, choosing to stay is only a limited option as the hospital is due to close soon anyway. This will mean that the familiar things will slowly be disappearing from his life as people move to their new situations. In a short period of time the hospital will no longer represent the place he now considers as home. It is important that George is made aware of these consequences, and the probability that someone else will take up the move he has on offer. However, in seeking to develop informed refusal it is important that the practitioner avoids anything which could amount to coercion as this invalidates the basis of informed choice.

The requirements of informed choice

The discussion of informed choice now focuses upon the conditions necessary to ensure that any choice made by a person is in fact an informed one. White (1989) argues that to be valid a person's consent must be given subject to the following conditions: 'To be valid, a consent must be given by a person who has received all relevant information, is competent, and has not been coerced into agreement or refusal' (White 1989: 6).

The first condition, that of relevant information, has provided the basis for much of the discussion above. This demonstrated that information is conveyed in a number of different ways, including discussions, the use of various media and experiential methods. It is important that information should be conveyed in the way most appropriate to each individual. Recent work on the development of methods designed to enable people with severe learning disabilities to articulate their opinions and evaluations has demonstrated the benefits of this approach in the promotion of informed choice (Flynn 1989, Whittaker *et al.* 1991). However, it has also demonstrated the need for much more work in this area.

The remaining conditions for informed choice relate to competence and coercion. They raise important questions for practice such as how a person with learning disability comes to be considered competent or incompetent; how that judgement is justified and recorded; and what methods practitioners use when seeking to support people in their choices. This involves a consideration of the concept of power.

Of all the issues discussed so far, that of competence is probably the most controversial. In the majority of the adult population competence is assumed upon the attainment of adult status. This status is defined not in terms of the demonstration of particular skills but solely by the achievement of a certain age, in Britain the age of 18 (Patterson 1978). The question of competence in relation to people with learning disabilities, however, smacks of paternalism. It is defined neither by age nor by law. Although Gunn argues that 'There is no legal decision that a person who is mentally handicapped is necessarily incapable of making treatment and care decisions' (Gunn 1985: 70), the fiduciary relationsahip places the question of competence within the duty of the practitioner.

The question then is: how do practitioners determine competence? This is a highly complex area which involves a series of judgements. For example, a person may be competent to perform one particular task and not competent to perform another. This is true of people generally. It is also the case that competence can vary over time; for example, anxiety or unfamiliar circumstances can influence a person's ability to perform a task, or to make a decision. And, as was pointed out earlier, decisions about options involving major life decisions have complex and unpredictable outcomes. Davis and Underwood provide the following analysis of the process of judging competence:

> Assessing competence becomes a process which culminates in a judgement. A judgement about competence is based upon (1) context of a specific task; (2) relevant abilities; (3) stability and variability of abilities; and (4) degree or extent of the relevant abilities.
>
> (Davis and Underwood 1989: 272)

Whatever judgement is made, it is essential for the practitioner to document fully the process of decision-making. This relates both to informed consent (Hollowell and Eldridge 1989, Scott 1991), and to informed refusal (Henry 1990, Weiss 1990). Documentation is important because it makes explicit both the judgements that have been made with respect to particular circumstances, and the basis for those judgements. There is also the issue that in human services, changes in people's lives or other choices they have made often require the reaffirmation of informed consent to a particular intervention (Weiss 1990, Scott 1991).

In the case of George, the question of competence may arise over his ability to choose to cross roads. In respect to context we can establish that George makes decisions to cross roads in his various journeys from the hospital to visit his friends or to go to the shops. This decision is made in the familiar context of his home town. The issue here would be to ensure that George, when faced with a similar type of road in the area to which he is considering moving, did not experience anxiety or other difficulties arising from the unfamiliar or different context which then affected his competence. The second issue is that of relevant abilities. Here it can be seen that George has the skills to negotiate the roads.

The third issue questions whether this ability is stable or if there are known circumstances when George's ability is impaired. For example, George may suffer from bouts of dizziness which would impair his competence with respect to crossing roads. Alternatively, he may rely upon certain aids such as glasses or a hearing appliance to maintain his competence. The final issue relates to the degree of the relevant abilities. Here the question would concern whether George can transfer his abilities to cross the road from the town roads to a more complex range of roads. For example, has he the competence to cross a dual carriageway, or use a zebra crossing when he is used to pelican crossings?

This now brings the discussion to the question of what tests are available where there is doubt or concern over the competence of an individual to make an informed choice. This question provides a difficult dilemma for the practitioner committed to the promotion of informed choice. Just what can be done when faced with a situation where the person is choosing a course of action which may cause considerable distress or even harm either to themselves or others.

Davis and Underwood (1989) discuss two possible tests. The first, which they refer to as the objective test, is derived from the reasonable person test discussed earlier. Here the subjective understanding of the person is not seen as the determining factor in the validity of informed choice, rather it is that person's general ability to function in comparison with a hypothetical person who is considered as being objectively reasonable. The second test, which they refer to as the subjective test, is based upon the person's actual understanding of the implications of their informed choice. Here the fact that a person is psychotic, severely mentally incapacitated or drugged, is viewed as irrelevant to the validity of that person's consent. This second test is argued to be very difficult to verify in practice (Davis and Underwood 1989).

The problems with these tests of competence are further complicated by another issue raised by the same authors. In relation to the practitioner's role they ask the following question, 'should the nurse be involved in determinations regarding mental competence and in the process of obtaining informed consent?' (Davis and Underwood 1989: 272).

One strategy that has been used to assist in this process of assessing competence is the use of a third person, such as a guardian or a citizen advocate. However, as Thorpe (1989) argues, this may only act to violate the principle of self-determination. Brennan makes a similar point, 'But the involvement of a third person does not restore autonomy but simply transfers it to someone else' (Brennan 1989: 48). There is also the problem of the legal principle when a third person is used in the attempt to establish informed consent. Here the advice of the Medical Protection Society is quite clear: regardless of the degree of incapacitation, a guardian or other third person cannot provide consent on behalf of a person over the age of 18 years (Medical Protection Society 1988).

The third requirement for informed choice is that of preventing coercion. However, the promotion of this condition is difficult because of the subtle ways in which it can take place. Friendly words of encouragement in respect of a particular option may be seen as coercive. This is especially true in environments that encourage compliance, such as hospitals (Gostin 1982). The same could be argued for residential homes, training centres and schools, as well as certain personal relationships where there is a clear imbalance of power. Arnstein (1969), in a model of power relations, identifies the power relationship in partnership as sharing, while those of therapy are associated with manipulation and non-participation.

In terms of the practitioner–client relationship this poses questions regarding the ways a person's experiences might be manipulated to ensure the choice or refusal of a particular intervention. The subtlety of this manipulation may be such that the practitioner is unaware of doing it. This situation can arise when the beliefs and values of the practitioner influence the opportunities that they facilitate for a particular person. It demonstrates the need for practitioners to be aware of their values if they are to avoid unintentional manipulative practices (White 1989). A case might be where a practitioner with strong moral views against pre-marital sexual relations sought to persuade a client not to set up home with his or her partner before marriage.

INFORMED CHOICE AND RISK

The final section considers the idea of risk and its management in circumstances where a person's growth could be enhanced through the exercise of a particular choice. In particular contexts, or as a result of particular desires, people may express the wish to bring a certain degree of risk into their lives. In these circumstances it may be difficult to establish that all the 'elements of informed choice' have been provided or the attendant 'requirements' satisfied. The size or the nature of the risk may also vary considerably from person to person. It may involve the potential of physical harm to the person or to others, or to property. On the other hand it may have the potential for emotional hurt or embarrassment. Alternatively, it may be a financial risk such as betting on a horse or buying a flat.

However, if practitioners are to act in ways which promote

autonomy, and in ways which recognise the potential of risk to the dignity of the person, then they have to establish methods of working with risk. They also have to identify the risks they as practitioners are taking. This requires that in the first place the practitioner consider carefully ways in which the risk can be reduced. Second, there is a need to document carefully the judgements that are made and the reasons for those judgements. This should include any dissenting views.

Examples of reducing risk might be as follows. There is a growing acknowledgement of the potential benefits for growth in challenging outdoor activities (Rose 1993). With respect to reducing risk it would be essential for a person wishing to go rock climbing to be properly dressed and accompanied by a qualified instructor. On the other hand, in the case of a person with a developing sexual relationship reducing risk might involve offering help and advice promoting sexual health. It should always be remembered that informed choice is a process and, likewise, so is the management of risk. For example, a person wishing to make a parachute jump practises ways of falling from steadily increasing heights before going for the real jump. In the same way people need opportunity to evaluate choices at many different stages before committing themselves to a decision. This idea of stages is one way in which both the 'elements' of and 'requirements' for informed choice can be managed through a developmental sequence.

SUMMARY

This chapter has discussed the concept of informed choice in relation to working with people with learning disability. The aim has been to establish the principles of informed choice and to focus on their implications for practice. The early part of the discussion drew upon philosophical concepts in order to establish the proposition that the debate involves moral and ethical commitments between human beings. This identified the ideas of autonomy and personal growth, and established the obligation we have to others to promote self-determination. This was contrasted with paternalism and the way in which this can be seen as a failure to act morally, with the consequence that dignity of person is denied. These ideas of obligation were then connected to the relationship between practitioners and their clients through the concept of the fiduciary relationship.

The practice of informed choice was shown to be a process

involving both time and education. First, the 'elements' which constitute the basis for informed choice were identified. This required delineation of the proposed intervention, the risks and benefits associated with that intervention, and alternatives which would deliver a similar or equivalent outcome. It also raised the question of informed refusal. Second, 'requirements' for informed choice relating to information, competence and coercion were discussed and set in the context of practice.

The final section considered risk: how this is related to the dignity and growth of the person, how it can be managed and the implications for practice.

KEY POINTS

Autonomy	**Foreseeable risk**
Beneficence	**Information**
Choice	**Informed consent**
Citizen advocate	**Informed refusal**
Coercion	**Personhood**
Competence	**Professionalism**
Duty	**Risk**
Fiduciary relationship	**Self-determination**

REFERENCES

Arnstein, S. (1969) 'A ladder of citizen participation', *Journal of the American Institute of Planners* 85(4): 215–24.

Brennan, A. (1989) 'Clinicians' conundrum', *Nursing Times* 85(20): 48–9.

Chappell, A.L. (1992) 'Towards a sociological critique of the normalisation principle', *Disability, Handicap and Society* 7(1): 35–51.

Coy, J.A. (1989) 'Autonomy-based informed consent: ethical implications for patient noncompliance', *Physical Therapy* 69(10): 826–33.

Crawley, B. (1988) *The Growing Voice*, London: V.I.A.

Croft, S. and Beresford, P. (1990) *From Paternalism to Participation. Involving People in Social Services*, London: Open Services Project and Joseph Rowntree Foundation.

Cushing, M. (1991) 'Demystifying informed consent', *American Journal of Nursing* 91(11): 17–19.

Davis, A.J. and Underwood, P.R. (1989) 'The competency quagmire: clarification of the nursing perspective concerning the issues of competence and informed consent', *International Journal of Nursing Studies* 26(3): 271–9.

Fiesta, J. (1991) 'Informed consent process – whose legal duty?', *Nursing Management* 22(1): 17–18.

Flynn, M. (1989) *Independent Living for People with Mental Handicap: 'A Place of my Own'*, London: Cassell Education.

Gorovitz, S. (1982) *Doctor's Dilemma: Moral Conflict and Medical Care*, New York: Macmillan Publishing Co.

Gostin, L.O. (1982) 'Psychosurgery: a hazardous and unestablished treatment', *Journal of Social Welfare Law* 4(2): 83–95.

Gunn, M. (1985) 'The law and mental handicap: consent to treatment', *Mental Handicap* 13: 70–2.

Haber, J.G. (1985) 'Patients, agents and informed consent', *Journal of Law and Health* 1(1): 43–59.

Henry, P.F. (1990) 'The doctrine of informed refusal', *Nurse Practitioner Forum* 1(2): 66–7.

Hollowell, E.E. and Eldridge, J.E. (1989) 'The nurse's role in informed consent', *The Journal of Practical Nursing* 9: 28–31.

Marsh, B.T. (1990) 'Informed consent – help or hindrance', *Journal of the Royal Society of Medicine*, vol. 83, 1990: 603–5.

Medical Protection Society (1988) *Consent; Confidentiality; Disclosure of Medical Records*, London: Medical Protection Society.

O'Brien, J. (1987) 'A guide to life-style planning; using the activities catalog to integrate services and natural support systems', in B. Wilcox and G.T. Bellamy (eds), *A Comprehensive Guide to the Activities Catalog. An Alternative Curriculum for Youth and Adults with Severe Disabilities*, Baltimore, Maryland: Paul Brooks Publishing.

Oliver, M. (1990) *The Politics of Disablement*, Basingstoke: Macmillan Educational.

Patterson, R.W.K. (1978) *Values, Education and the Adult*, Boston, Massachusetts: Routledge & Kegan Paul.

Rose, S. (1993) 'Integrated leisure activities', in M. Todd and P. Brigden, *Concepts in Community Care For People with a Learning Disability*, Basingstoke: Macmillan Educational.

Scott, R.W. (1991) 'Informed consent', *Clinical Management* 11(3): 12–14.

Smith, C.K. (1990) 'Legal review: informed consent – a shift from paternalism to self-determination?', *Topics in Health Record Management* 9: 71–5.

Thorpe, L. (1989) 'Informed decision making', *Nursing* 3(42): 16–19.

Weiss, F.S. (1990) 'The right to refuse: informed consent and the psychological nurse', *Journal of Psychological Nursing* 28(8): 25–30.

White, B. (1989) 'Ethical issues surrounding informed consent: Part iii. The crucial role of nursing in insuring valid consent', *Urological Nursing* July–September: 6–9.

Whittaker, A., Gardener, S. and Kershaw, J. (1991) *Service Evaluation By People With Learning Difficulties*, London: The King's Fund Centre.

Chapter 5

Empowerment: issues, tensions and conflicts

Tony Gilbert

INTRODUCTION

The aim of this chapter is to explore the concept of empowerment in the context of working with people with a learning disability. Empowerment will be identified as a complex idea which, in contemporary debates over welfare policy, has entered the professional jargon of health and welfare professionals, managers, politicians and administrators. Empowerment is not a recent idea, but previously it was mainly articulated by those dependent upon welfare services, such as disabled people. It was part of their demand for a more effective response to their needs from agencies such as personal social services and local health services. Disabled people, along with other users of welfare services, argued that these services ignored their real needs, imposing professional definitions of need instead. This had the effect of compounding disability by eroding the control disabled people had over their own lives and brought with it the experience of powerlessness as they became increasingly dependent upon welfare professionals and the services they controlled.

The adoption of the concept of empowerment by welfare professionals, managers and politicians has meant that a complex and ambiguous idea has been included within professional discourse in a way that ignores its essentially problematic nature. As a result there is a danger of losing empowerment's potential to provide a radical alternative to a professional practice which can be paternalistic and dependency-creating. The objectives of this chapter are therefore to clarify the nature of empowerment, to identify it as having both costs and benefits for those involved, and to discuss the ethics of empowerment. An appreciation of these aspects is necessary if professional practice is to be credible in any claims it makes of being empowering, or alternatively, in its ability to recognise professional practices that are dependency-creating.

The following approach is adopted. First, the concept of empowerment is explored and identified as having both psychological and political dimensions. In doing this it is essential to locate empowerment and empowering practices within the community, that is, within the social relationships and political structures through which people live their lives, for these represent the means through which problems are defined and resources identified.

The second section of the chapter then defines empowerment as the achievement of a 'participatory competence', which is the result of a developmental process. This refers on the one hand to the acquisition of a psychological outlook by the person which challenges negative self-images, low self-esteem, and feelings of powerlessness. On the other hand, and at the same time, it refers to the acquisition of social and political skills necessary to challenging the processes of definition and decision-making within the community.

The third section considers processes for acquiring skills for 'participatory competence'. These are referred to as 'social technologies'. The definition of a social technology covers a wide range of activities, the condition being that it should be possible for other people to replicate the same activity in different contexts. The important point is to separate specific strategies for the development of skills intended to facilitate 'participatory competence' from the particular relationships that develop between individuals. This section is illustrated by a fictitious case study which is also used as a basis for the fourth section. This involves a discussion of the ethical considerations implicit in working towards empowerment. These arise as a result of the costs and benefits a disabled person may experience through empowerment and which may, in turn, have implications for other people close to the person, including professional practitioners.

EMPOWERMENT: CLARIFYING THE CONCEPT

The problem of definition

The aim from the outset is to identify the ambiguous nature of the concept of empowerment. This ambiguity has arisen, in part, due to the articulation of the term within different, and often competing, discourses. The term has been used in a variety of different ways in different contexts, many of which can be demonstrated to be inappropriate. For example, the 1990s has seen the term used in relation to providing information. This falls a long way short of the definition of 'participatory competence' that is used here. Professionals have been active in exploiting this ambiguity and empowerment has become an influential jargon word in health and welfare services.

The definition of empowerment is further complicated by the fact that it has found its way into the political demands of the Left, Right, and Centre of British politics. In this way it can provide a central idea in potentially competing movements calling for either welfare consumerism or user participation. Its appeal originates, as Adams (1990) points out, in the long tradition of self-help in British welfare, which is strongly linked to philanthropy and nineteenth-century middle-class attitudes towards the 'deserving' and 'undeserving' poor. These held that charity was morally harmful to both the individual and to society. Similar viewpoints continue to be expressed today in the continuing influence of the New Right upon Conservative ministers and policy-makers (Loney *et al.* 1991: 7).

Adams goes on to identify four perspectives which seek to explain the growth of self-help. These are: a traditionalist perspective that argues that people have always engaged in individual or collective self-help; a functionalist perspective that argues that self-help arises due to gaps in the services supplied by professionals; a liberal perspective that proposes self-help as an alternative to professional views. Finally, there is a radical perspective that mounts a critique of social policy and professional practice as dehumanising, with the consequence of alienating people from their communities. Here self-help is viewed as taking place within collective action, and is seen as a means towards greater personal autonomy and democracy. Each of these perspectives, in turn, sets out its own version of the relationship between the individual or group and wider socio-political structures.

The attraction for professional practice

Following on from the argument above, the question arises as to what function this adoption of empowerment serves for professionals. Mullender and Ward (1991) point out that to argue that practice is empowering is to appear progressive and morally superior. It has the effect of placing practitioners in a position where they are beyond challenge or criticism. They argue that it is used despite the fact that it masks inherent tensions. Its use in professional jargon is such that 'It acts as a social "aerosol", covering up the disturbing smell of conflict and conceptual division' (Mullender and Ward 1991: 1). In this context empowerment is being used to protect professional practice from scrutiny.

At the same time the ambiguity of empowerment provides a means of avoiding clarification and resolution of tensions in the practice of professionals. For example, what exact form or forms of practice can be demonstrated as empowering? Here Adams (1990) argues that there is a lack of readily identifiable guidelines for practitioners. The concept of empowerment inevitably raises questions about the power relationship between disabled people and their immediate carers, but it also raises questions about the relationship between disabled people, professionals, managers and politicians. It points to the political nature of these relationships, and, in turn, to the tensions that will inevitably arise between those with power and those who seek empowerment. This is true regardless of whether people are seeking empowerment for themselves or for others. There is therefore a crucial need to acknowledge the personal as political as the value base for a professional practice which can truly claim to be empowering (Mullender and Ward 1991: 6).

Mullender and Ward go on to identify the dilemma implicit in practice which aims to be empowering. This arises because empowerment has to be understood as having implications for both the person or group, and the professional worker. They point out that in adopting a form of practice which aims to be empowering, professionals need to recognise that there is no position of neutrality: 'Once the impossibility of neutrality is recognised, in that it colludes with oppression, we would argue, social action becomes inevitable' (Mullender and Ward 1991: 16). This in turn raises issues over the degree to which professional workers have real control over the nature of their practice. It also identifies the inevitable conflict they will experience.

Identifying outcomes

The ambiguity in providing a definition arises not only because empowerment is articulated within different discourses, or because of the lack of guidelines for professional practice. It is further complicated by the difficulty in establishing what empowerment is or when it has occurred. Rappaport (1981) provides the following definition of empowerment: 'Enhancing the possibilities for people to control their own lives'. The problem here then becomes one of defining what exactly this means for individual people. He later extends the definition by including both subjective and objective criteria:

> For some people the mechanism of empowerment may lead to a sense of control; for others it may lead to actual control, the practical power to affect their own lives.
>
> (Rappaport 1984: 3)

Rappaport then seeks to further highlight the outcomes of empowerment by defining them in the negative, that is, by referring to powerlessness:

> Empowerment is easy to define in its absence: powerlessness, real or imagined; learned helplessness; alienation; loss of a sense of control over one's life. It is more difficult to define positively only because it takes on different forms in different people and contexts.
>
> (Rappaport 1984: 3)

This is not to argue that it was inappropriate to define empowerment in a negative way, rather that the consequence is that it leaves both the outcomes and process of empowerment as being specific to individuals, and relative to their social circumstances. Defining it negatively also runs the risk of further adding to the ambiguity of the concept.

In order to quantify when empowerment has occurred, Rappaport suggests that the answer may lie in identifying parameters, that is:

> Under what conditions do we find people reporting a sense of control over their own lives? We need not limit our questions to particular contents of control. It may include political, economic, interpersonal, psychological, or spiritual control.
>
> (Rappaport 1984: 4)

Empowerment is therefore a concept which relates both to people's personal attributes and to their social circumstances; it has psychological and political dimensions. It is important to identify the multi-dimensional nature of empowerment as this provides the ambiguity which often allows only one of its dimensions to be considered, that is, the psychological dimension.

Adams (1990) extends this problem of definition further. First, he identifies the possibility of empowerment for both individuals and groups. Second, he implies that a differential experience of empowerment is possible within different aspects of people's lives. Finally, he introduces the concept of 'quality of life', without making it clear exactly what he means by this. He argues that empowerment:

> can be defined as the process by which individuals, groups and/or communities become able to take control of their circumstances and achieve their own goals, thereby being able to work towards maximizing the quality of their lives. The process of empowerment operates at the levels of the individual, group, family, organisation and community, and also in different sectors of people's lives.
>
> (Adams 1990: 43)

Before moving to a concept analysis of empowerment it is useful to summarise the argument so far. Empowerment is a multi-dimensional concept, and its practice creates tensions due to the fact that it involves a process of personal change. This change takes place both within the person and in the social relationships that person has with others. The critical issue in empowerment is that people cannot be separated from their social environment: 'Empowerment is therefore not independent of relationships with those who provide care and with the wider community in which they live' (Brown and Ringma 1989: 253).

Empowerment has to be considered as a dynamic process. It involves a complex inter-relationship of change which will have costs and benefits to the person, as well as the possibility of unintentional outcomes.

A concept analysis

The previous section has demonstrated that the concept of empowerment raises difficulties in definition and tensions in its application. Kieffer offers the following insight into this problem: 'While the idea of empowerment is intuitively appealing for both theory and practice, its applicability has been limited by continued conceptual ambiguity' (Kieffer 1984: 9).

This section will seek to establish the conceptual basis of empowerment in two ways. First, by identifying the relationship between people and their psychological and political selves. Second, by describing a developmental process which leads from powerlessness to empowerment.

Katz (1984) identifies the problem of empowerment as one which arises from the very nature of contemporary Western industrialised society. He argues that resources and power itself are commodities that have particular values, and that such valued resources are scarce. In turn, it is this scarcity that determines their value. The implication of this is that individuals or communities must compete for access to these resources. The result is to promote individual accumulation and a resistance to sharing. People and communities are told to place their trust in the market as a means of fairly distributing these scarce resources, despite continuing evidence of inequality. Therefore, as power is a valued commodity there will be a resistance to empowering forms of practice as these imply the redistribution of power from the powerful to the powerless. This point is crucial to the debate over welfare services when one considers the claims of professions for the power to accredit and control particular bodies of knowledge, to license the practice of particular forms of skill, and to define needs.

Katz locates the problem of empowerment in social relations, that is, in the norms and values which govern the ways people behave, and the practices that social institutions promote. In Western society questions over empowerment are often framed in terms such as: 'How do we empower "those" people and still reserve for ourselves all the resources we have now?' (Katz 1984: 203).

Empowerment therefore implies a fundamental change in the social relationships between the powerful and powerless. However, these relationships go beyond individual disabled people, professionals and so on. They are institutionalised in welfare practices and reinforced by social policy. Katz argues that 'Empowerment is not limited to or identifiable with individuals, it becomes a resource beyond the self. It occurs across individuals and within communities' (Katz 1984: 204).

In identifying power as a scarce and valued resource it can be seen that those with power develop subtle ways of oppression through becoming 'experts'. These experts, possibly with the best of intentions, create circumstances where the initial reliance upon their expertise and knowledge continues. The effect is that 'Those who seek power continue to direct the process of empowerment, and those who seek to become empowered continue to look outside themselves for advice' (Katz 1984: 205).

Katz, in establishing empowerment as a characteristic of societies, provides two essential elements to this process of concept analysis. First, in locating empowerment as a characteristic of societies he moves away from views of empowerment that seek to locate it as a purely psychological attribute. This has important implications for all those who claim to be working in empowering ways. He argues that 'Empowerment is an actual as well as perceived sense of power, an observable effect on socio-political structures as well as a subjective experience' (Katz 1984: 205). In doing so, he rejects the propositions of humanistic psychologists such as Rogers (1979), who have stressed the importance of the perceived sense of power in the process of human meaning-making. Katz argues that:

> Rogers would establish the possibility of empowerment as a limitless resource if self understanding were the only obstacle. But his relative emphasis upon the perceived sense rather than the actual exercise of power, and upon personal experience rather than social structures, does not attend sufficiently to socio-political obstacles to self understanding and especially to expressing that understanding in action.
>
> (Katz 1984: 205)

Empowerment involves new ways of making sense of experience. This requires the establishment of new relationships between people and the sociopolitical structures they encounter that reflect this new consciousness.

Second, Katz locates the potential for empowerment within the community, which turns the focus towards the nature of particular communities and how their potential for empowerment might be maximised. The question then becomes one of how this potential for empowerment is released within communities. Katz argues that power need not be a limited resource and that strategies can be adopted which develop power. He continues by pointing to the work of Freire (1970), and his development of the concept of praxis as a demonstration of how power can expand. Praxis involves a process where the experience of direct action in confronting social oppression is linked with reflection to provide new understandings. These, in turn, produce new and more effective forms of social action. Freire argues that power can expand as people get together to identify the source of their oppression and take action to change the system.

The importance of focusing upon sociopolitical structures rather than solely psychological attributes is further reinforced by Rappaport (1984). Again he focuses upon the importance of particular communities, arguing that we need to develop an understanding of the naturally occurring helping systems that emerge in families, communities, and other social networks. For it is these that provide the psychological supports through which people find meaning in life. This understanding may then lead to more meaningful alternatives for those who do not fit in than the limited options developed by professionals. This point is echoed by Biegel:

> Why should we force clients to fit their problems into the frameworks professionals have created to meet their needs? Rather, we should discover how clients naturally solve their problems and meet their needs and then graft professional interventions onto this natural process.
>
> (Biegel 1984: 119)

This brings the discussion to another important principle in the analysis of empowerment, that is, the need to be critically aware of the relationship between the targets of empowerment and those working to support those individuals, groups or communities. Rappaport describes this relationship as follows:

> Empowerment may be the result of programmes designed by professionals, but more likely will be found in those circumstances where there is either true collaboration among professionals and the supposed beneficiaries, or in settings and under conditions where professionals are not the key actors.
>
> (Rappaport 1984: 4)

A further conceptual element is added to the analysis when the nature of solutions is considered, as there may be more than one solution. This then implies that each possible solution is likely to bring different combinations of costs and benefits. Rappaport highlights the paradoxical nature of problems in community life, and he points to the possibility that some proposed solutions may well be contradictory in that they are found in equally compelling opposites. He provides the following example:

> providing for the perceived needs of people may sometimes infringe upon their rights, and assuring right does not necessarily satisfy needs. In short, most social problems are more complex and involve interrelationships among opposites in such a fashion that there is no single solution which 'solves' the problem. Consequently, the method of investigation required, because of the very nature of social problems, is

a dialectical one, governed by divergent, rather than convergent thinking.

(Rappaport 1984: 2)

A further element to this concept analysis is provided by Hess (1984) who argues, 'As empowerment is a dynamic, it must have negative as well as positive features' (Hess 1984: 229). This could be seen for example in the actions of a person who, in seeking more control of his or her life, may alienate and lose the support of paternalistic colleagues or neighbours. Therefore empowerment may entail costs as well as benefits, or costs before benefits. Also, for many people facing social oppression, survival is a full-time occupation; therefore seeking to become involved just adds to the burden.

Summary

Empowerment can be seen to be a complex multi-dimensional concept which contains many ambiguities. Its links with the idea of self-help have led to its articulation within a range of political and professional discourses. However, this ambiguity has led to considerable confusion and misuse of the term. In providing a concept analysis of empowerment the following elements have been identified: power and empowerment have to be located within the sociopolitical structure of a particular society; empowerment has political as well as psychological dimensions; the focus for empowerment working has to be in the person's community, and this has to address the nature of professional solutions; the solutions to issues of empowerment are dynamic, complex, and quite probably contradictory.

THE PROCESS OF EMPOWERMENT: TOWARDS PARTICIPATORY COMPETENCE

The first part of this section takes the discussion of empowerment on to a consideration of the process through which individuals may pass, and the development of the psychological and the political aspects of their lives. The second part considers strategies, the so-called 'social technologies' that may enable the achievement of 'participatory competence'.

The experience of powerlessness

Kieffer describes empowerment as a long-term process of adult learning and development which has the purpose of achieving what he describes as 'multi-dimensional participatory competence' (Kieffer 1984: 9). In this, empowerment is conceptualised as an inter-active and highly subjective relationship between individuals and their environment. Powerlessness, on the other hand, is seen as trapping people into a cycle of victimisation and self-blame. This condition was described by Freire as one where individuals consider themselves as object rather than subject: 'As such the individual alienates him/herself from participation in the construction of social reality' (Freire 1970).

Powerlessness is the state where individuals hold an expectancy that their own behaviour will not, and cannot, effect or determine access to the resources or opportunities they desire. This, in turn, leads to a condition where people no longer even consider such opportunities. They accept that their condition is 'natural' and therefore beyond the possibility of change. The result of powerlessness can be seen in the feelings of alienation and distrust that are expressed by many with long-term experiences of welfare services. This powerlessness can be measured in the material conditions of people's lives, that is, in their exclusion from social and community resources, and their economic vulnerability.

Kieffer goes on to identify the role social institutions within the community have in reinforcing and compounding these feelings of powerlessness. He argues: 'Major public institutions ie: schools, church, the press, and local government, function as partners in the suppression of individual initiative. Their intimidation is especially intense in relation to the experience of economic insecurity' (Kieffer 1984: 16).

This highlighting of the economic aspect links with the earlier comments of Rappaport (1984) identifying power as a commodity within a market-orientated society. It is here that the link between the material conditions of a person's life and the psychological aspect is made. People, either as individuals or as communities, find themselves unable to protect themselves from the ongoing experience of marginalisation and discrimination. This arises as people's past experience influences their present ongoing behaviour through the establishment of a particular cognitive framework. Kieffer argues that: 'While not seen as unilaterally imposed upon the individual by his/her environment, powerlessness is viewed as an experience embedded in and reinforced by the fabric of such institutions' (Kieffer 1984: 14).

From powerlessness to empowerment

At this point in the discussion it is useful to recognise that empowerment is not achieved merely by recognising the feeling of powerlessness and oppression, although this recognition is essential to its achievement. Instead, empowerment has to be conceptualised as a long-term process which involves the acquisition of political skills and insights, the objective of which is the condition of participatory competence referred to earlier. Kieffer summarises this point as follows: 'Empowerment then assumes a dual meaning. It refers both to a longitudinal dynamic of development and to attainment of a set of insights and abilities best characterised as "participatory competence" ' (Kieffer 1984: 18–19).

Kieffer offers a developmental model of the process of moving from powerlessness to empowerment. This is described as an ordered and progressive development from sociopolitical infancy to adulthood. It relates to the acquisition of a particular psychological outlook which first recognises the possibility of particular resources and opportunities, and second includes the necessary skills to articulate this outlook to others. This work is based upon a study of emerging grass-roots activists in community organisations. He describes a process of development involving four stages through which people move. However, there is no reason to assume that this model cannot be successfully applied in other areas of welfare. As with the earlier reference to the costs and benefits of empowerment, Kieffer points to the tensions that the person will experience from the initiation of the empowerment process. He identifies this dissonance as essential as it motivates personal response, and once again it highlights the dynamic nature of empowerment: 'In the struggle towards empowerment, conflict and growth are inextricably intertwined. It is essential that individuals continue to experience conflict to sustain their emergence' (Kieffer 1984: 25).

The implication of such a model of developmental stages is that the former stage has to be completed before the person can move successfully on to the next stage. However, Kieffer does seek to quantify these stages by setting minimum times within which each could be achieved. This provides a vivid reminder to those seeking to work in empowering ways of the long-term commitment required.

The first stage of the process is described as the 'era of entry' and as taking at least one year to achieve. It involves a critical event in the empowerment process, that is, a sense of personal violation. Kieffer explains that this has to be more than the daily experience of exploitation, as it has to include a direct threat to a person's well-being or dignity or that of the person's family. This then represents a fundamental shift in the psychological outlook referred to earlier where helplessness is accepted and the possibilities of particular opportunities are not even considered. In doing this the individual achieves a state of beginning to confront and engage the systems of authority and, through this, demystifying their power. Kieffer argues that moving through this initial phase 'demands especially that each individual alter his/her sense of relation to long established symbols and systems of authority' (Kieffer 1984: 19).

The second stage is referred to as the 'era of advancement' which Kieffer identifies with later childhood and which is viewed as taking at least one year. This stage sees the establishment of particular social relationships and a developing sociopolitical awareness.

The three major aspects of the empowering evolution in this phase are the centrality of a mentoring relationship, the enabling impact of supportive peer relationships within a collective organisational structure, and the cultivation of a more critical understanding of social and political relations.

(Kieffer 1984: 20)

In identifying the centrality of the mentoring relationship to this stage of development, Kieffer highlights a role for someone to support the individual through the empowerment process. This person is seen as a role model and mentor, providing emotional support and nurturing independent action and the development of unpractised political skills. The mentor is also an educator, demystifying the political process and negotiating new authority relationships.

Kieffer also highlights a process similar to that of Freire's concept of praxis, which involves the development of understanding through practical experience and reflection. He argues: 'Action informs understanding to the extent that individuals accept responsibility for their choices and engage in self critical reflection upon their efforts' (Kieffer 1984: 21). This implies that individuals must become involved in the real process of confronting their oppression, and that they must actively make choices and accept the responsibility for those choices. In this it can be demonstrated that participatory competence can only begin to be achieved through direct experience, and that choice and risk are central to this.

The establishment of a peer group also appears to be essential to the development of rudimentary political skills. The purpose of this group is to place conflicts into a political framework which seeks to identify the inter-connectedness of social, political and economic relations, rather than to provide emotional support, although its contribution to the latter function is recognised. The third stage of this developmental process is referred to as the 'era of incorporation'. This is likened to adolescence, and again a minimum of one year is given for its achievement. This stage involves the maturation of both psychological and political aspects of the person. Self-concept, strategic ability and critical comprehension are now such that the person can learn to confront the permanence and painfulness of institutional barriers to self-determination. This demands the development of leadership and organisational skills. However, there are continuing costs to the empowerment process, and these might be experienced differently according to gender: 'participants also are required to resolve the multiple role conflicts and social strains generated by enduring community involvement. This task is especially straining for women' (Kieffer 1984: 23). Kieffer reports that many of the participants in his study referred to this stage as 'growing up'. They described the need to resolve personal conflicts relating to self-esteem and self-confidence.

The final stage of this process, the 'era of commitment', is considered to be a more mature state of empowerment and it is likened to adulthood. In this stage participants continue to struggle to integrate new personal knowledge and skill into the reality and structure of their social worlds. This relates to a search for viable and personally meaningful ways of applying the skills and awareness gained through the developmental process.

This idea of a developmental process involving moving from powerlessness to empowerment has important implications for the theory and practice of empowerment. It implies that people have first to experience their oppression and to recognise it for what it is. Following this there is a long-term process of development that has emotional and time costs. Finally, and very importantly, people have to practise using their developing political skills. The reason for promoting empowerment is summarised by Kieffer as follows: 'The "preventative" impact of this model resides in the development of competences required to counteract the dehumanising and destructive social forces which underlie most human stress and dysfunction' (Kieffer 1984: 32).

SOCIAL TECHNOLOGIES: TOWARDS PARTICIPATORY COMPETENCE

Having considered both the concept of empowerment and the nature of the developmental process, it is now possible to consider practical strategies. These strategies can be used to promote transition and they provide the basis for a way of working by professionals to facilitate empowerment. These diverse forms of activity are described as social technologies which are defined in the following way: 'A social technology is a replicable set of procedures that is designed to produce an effect upon socially important behaviours of relevant participants under a variety of real life conditions' (Fawcett *et al.* 1984: 147).

The following case study is intended to facilitate the discussion of social technologies and the later discussion of ethical considerations with respect to the practice of empowerment.

Case study: Margaret Adams

Margaret Adams is 32 years old, and lives in a council house on an estate in a small Midlands town. Since her mother died four years ago, she has shared the house with her father, Dave. Margaret has one brother, James, who lives with his wife Avril and their two small children, Michael and Len, in an estate on the other side of town. Margaret also has a sister, Jean, who is a sergeant in the RAF and lives overseas. Margaret has always lived in the house where she is now living, and since leaving school at 19 she has been a 'trainee' at the local authority social education centre, which is in the next town. When the time came to leave school, Margaret's teacher told her that she would never be able to get a 'proper job' as she was 'educationally subnormal'. Now she is told she has 'a learning disability', although from Margaret's point of view she feels just the same. She used to enjoy going to the centre as it gave her the chance to meet her friends, particularly John. John is very special to Margaret and they describe themselves as being 'in love'.

However, about a year ago John got a job at the local hypermarket. This means that they see each other only in the evening, as John works at the weekend. Most of the time they see each other at Margaret's house so they have little privacy. John talks to Margaret about his job, about the money he earns, about being a member of the union, and about the mates he now has. He has also been telling Margaret that there are jobs at the hypermarket that she would be good at. Margaret is quite envious of John, although she is pleased that he enjoys his job, for her job at the centre pays very little. Also, it is quite clear that she isn't a member of staff, for although she has a clear set of tasks and is trusted to work in reception, she cannot leave the centre at lunchtime to go shopping without asking permission, nor is she allowed to use the staff toilets.

At home, Margaret performs most of the household tasks for her father. She shops, washes and irons, cleans and tidies, and helps prepare and cook the meals. Since her mother died Margaret has taken to 'caring for her father', and she will often limit her own activities by saying, 'I cannot go because Dad will need me to cook his tea' or, 'I better get home as I have to sort the ironing out'. Mr Adams doesn't ask or insist that Margaret is home. On the other hand he doesn't do anything to discourage her feelings of responsibility or her perception of his dependency.

Moreover, Mr Adams does not encourage Margaret to be more independent and he actively obstructs any development of the relationship between Margaret and John. His attitude tends to be that he and Margaret are all right as they are, and her relationship with John is purely a friendship, anything else would be beyond their understanding. The problem here for Margaret is that although John talks about them getting a flat together, he is tending to treat Margaret very similarly to the way her father does.

This general situation was one that Margaret tended to accept, although she often wished that she could be like her sister and brother and have her own home and a job. Sometimes she used to dream of having her own baby, but she would push these thoughts out of her mind telling herself not to be so silly. However it did tend to get her down at times. Once, when she went to the GP on her own, he had told her that she was depressed. This worried her greatly as somebody she knew at the centre had been depressed and had to go to hospital. It also made her feel angry as she felt that she was being blamed for things she had no control over.

Things began to change for Margaret after John had left the centre and got his job. There was a reorganisation of the centre and Margaret's job changed without her being asked. Then, a little later, Margaret went to her Life Plan meeting with the idea of asking about leaving and getting a job. She had been promised at the previous two meetings that her name was going to be put forward for a new work scheme that social services were running. However, when she got there nobody wanted to listen, instead the discussion focused upon her relationship with John. The meeting decided she needed counselling and sex education. Margaret wanted to tell them to mind their own business, but she didn't. Things finally came to a head when Margaret had the chance to go away for a holiday with John and some other friends at the centre.

A sense of personal violation

Earlier in this chapter, in the discussion of Kieffer's model of the development from powerlessness to empowerment, we noted the importance of a critical event in a person's life which will stimulate the development of the empowerment process. In Margaret's case the holiday provided this event. She was very excited at the prospect of the trip to Scotland. However, when she told her father he was far from enthusiastic. Mr Adams didn't tell Margaret that she couldn't go, instead he began a campaign of placing obstacles in her way, especially emotional obstacles. He began to play on his health, getting Margaret to telephone the health centre, claiming that he was unable to walk and had chest pains. In the end Margaret gave in and withdrew from the trip. John, on the other hand, continued with his plans and, from Margaret's point of view, he didn't seem to care that she would not be there.

The time came for the holiday and Margaret was left behind. She looked and felt really lonely. Mr Adams, seeing this, said that he would make up for her disappointment and he promised Margaret a good night out. However, when the time came, the night out was a disaster. The treat turned out to be a trip to the dog races, followed by a drink at the local. Mr Adams lost some money betting which put him in a bad mood. Following this he met some friends at the pub and totally ignored Margaret, and after getting quite drunk he invited his friends back to the house for a nightcap and a fish supper. Margaret found herself waiting on her father and his friends. Then, as they were all drinking, the TV was switched on for an 'adult' film. In front of all these people Mr Adams sent Margaret to bed.

Margaret felt bitter and angry, but more so than ever before. This time she felt that her dignity had been violated, and she was offended and deeply hurt. But at the same time Margaret was feeling confused; everything in her life focused around her being put upon by others, her father, people at the centre, social services, and John, who treated her in the same way as her father. The next day Margaret went to town to see Jenny Moore. Jenny had been a worker at the centre but she had now left to work in her own shop in the arcade. When she had been at the centre, Jenny had sought to encourage Margaret to strike out and to lead her own life. The importance of the 'mentoring' relationship is identified by Kieffer in his description of the second stage of development towards empowerment. Here this relationship can be seen to develop between Margaret and Jenny. Margaret trusted Jenny, and they shared a considerable rapport. They met and talked on a number of occasions over the next couple of weeks, but Margaret's feelings of oppression remained as strong.

Towards self-definition

Self-definition is linked to the sense of personal violation. It relates to the process of rejecting externally defined and controlling images that help to produce powerlessness. Margaret expressed her feelings of powerlessness to Jenny. She described her disappointment with her father, with John, with work, and she explained how she tended to accept things. Jenny felt that they needed to work in two ways: the first would focus upon Margaret's self-image, the second would focus upon her relationship with others. Following a series of discussions, Jenny and Margaret agreed that Jenny would assist Margaret to construct her own history using her own definitions and feelings. As this developed, Margaret began to include things personal to herself, photographs, drawings and paintings, a couple of poems, and knicknacks that were important to her.

In this first instance, social technologies can be seen to involve strategies that establish for the person or group a history, art, literature, music or poetry, or other forms of creative expression that provide self-valuations that challenge those that are externally defined. The importance of this is described by Hill Collins (1990), in the context of black women's empowerment: 'By persisting in the journey towards self definition we are changed, and this change empowers us' (Hill Collins 1990: 221). In relation to the discussion of empowerment in working with people with a learning disability, the anthology *Know Me as I am* (Atkinson and Williams 1990) provides an interesting range of examples of work towards self-definition. In the context of self-definition, the change in self-valuation contributes to an epistemological debate which creates new ways of considering the 'truth'. This, in turn, creates new knowledge about the potentially empowering experiences of individuals and groups.

Developing supportive peer relations

In conjunction with the importance of the mentoring relationship, Kieffer identifies two other essential facets of this second stage towards empowerment. These are the importance of supportive peer relations within an organised structure, and the cultivation of a critical awareness of political and social relations. Here Fawcett *et al.* (1984) point out the importance of social technologies being compatible with the resources and values of the people or communities involved: 'Such technologies are particularly useful if they are designed to be inexpensive, effective, decentralised, flexible, sustainable, simple and compatible with existing customs, beliefs and values' (Fawcett *et al.* 1984: 147). The challenge here is for professionals or other people involved in empowerment working to recognise the characteristics of communities. For, as Biegel (1984) argued, professionals have tended to operate with little knowledge or understanding of community ties or informal networks.

With regard to developing supportive peer relations, Jenny discussed with Margaret the possibility of joining the women's group run by the local adult education centre. Margaret agreed and she soon found that she shared many of the experiences and frustrations of the other women in the group. She also learned some assertiveness skills and she started to feel good about herself in a way that she had not experienced previously. Jenny also agreed that she would provide support to Margaret at other times, the first opportunity being her Life Plan meeting. On these occasions the aim was not for Jenny to speak for Margaret, rather to provide her with guidance and feedback regarding the way her participatory skills were developing.

Developing a critical awareness

A further development in Margaret's life occurred at the suggestion of some of the people who used the centre, following a discussion with a local advocacy worker. This involved the setting up of a group within the centre to discuss issues of interest and concern. This presented the possibility of developing a supportive peer group. The advantages of such groups has been described by Crawley (1988). Jenny and some other people agreed to support the group by helping to facilitate the meetings which took place in the centre in the evening. The following section outlines a groupwork process which has been demonstrated to facilitate empowerment.

One particular social technology that has been described as empowering is described by Mullender and Ward (1989) as 'self-directed groupwork'. This aims to empower group members through a process where they set their own goals for extended change. The first stage of this process involves workers in establishing an agreed and explicit value position. It is from this value position that practice must flow. Mullender and Ward argue that other group work models leave their value base to be implied from observation, or they claim a philosophy and then allow scope for the practitioner to use the model without a conscious awareness of the values it implies. Self-directed groupwork aims to ensure open planning right from the start, with as much responsibility as possible being handed over to the group.

The avoidance of initial planning stages attended only by workers aims to avoid a predetermined agenda. This enables the achievement of the central aim of this method which is 'unfettered goal setting'. Here group members set their own goals. This does not mean that workers do not start out with a purpose, for this purpose is the general aim of empowering members. Furthermore, and linking with the political nature of empowerment, it is essential that workers do not shut out possibilities of moving on from common experience to broader social issues. However, this does not mean that the group will not require skilled facilitation, especially in the initial stages.

Another principle is that of 'non-selected membership'. Here Mullender and Ward argue that referrals tend to set particular criteria, therefore in self-directed groupwork members should either choose to come, belong to a natural group, or have the potential to form a group identity. Another important idea is that the group should have an 'open-ended length', that is, the group should decide its timespan rather than this being related to the commitment of workers. Here it is important that workers do not under-estimate the length of time needed before a group can become member-led. This requires a long-term commitment from workers, or it may involve a team of workers. Some appreciation of the time period can be drawn from Kieffer's developmental model.

Further organisational issues, such as the time and place of meetings, aim to utilise the way people tend to meet naturally:

> It is important for self-directed groupwork to tap into the natural dynamics of group interaction as far as possible because this is what the workers are there to facilitate; they are often not trying to create a new group identity from scratch but to enhance what already exists in embryo at least.
>
> (Mullender and Ward 1989: 17)

For example, groups from a day centre, such as the one Margaret attends, or a residential home, may have a natural dynamic and that group can then meet in its natural everyday setting.

The internal conduct of the group is also critical to the success of the group as 'self directed groupwork is grounded in the notion of a working agreement between workers and members' (Mullender and Ward 1989: 19). Some of these matters need to be established early in the group's life. These include issues of confidentiality between members and workers, between the group and the outside world, and between individuals and any external agency from whom they may be receiving help. Beyond this, however, group rules must be set by the group as they discover what rules they require.

This latter point is further reinforced by Mullender and Ward, who point out that workers should not place matters on to the agenda and they should only refer to matters as they arise within the group. However, they argue that:

> As a group develops over time however, members increasingly offer each other this support both inside and outside the group and, where they feel something is out of their scope, will often help the person concerned to seek appropriate sources of help outside of the group.
>
> (Mullender and Ward 1989: 23)

In seeking to promote a member-centred approach to empowerment, Mullender and Ward point to the importance of the implicit and explicit intentions and purposes of leadership. Decisions, and the responsibility for these, must fall fully upon the group. If this is left to default, it will work to reinforce rather than to question dominant social values.

ETHICAL CONSIDERATIONS FOR EMPOWERMENT STRATEGIES

The aim of this final section is to illustrate some of the ethical considerations essential to the choice of empowerment as the goal of professional practice. To summarise the case study: first, it would appear that Margaret has experienced the 'personal violation' that Kieffer argues to be essential. In experiencing this Margaret has begun to reject her ideas of helplessness. Second, the possibilities for mentorship are there in the relationship with Jenny, which is also facilitating the process of self-definition, while the women's group and the advocacy group both provide possibilities for peer group support, and for the development of a critical awareness. Finally, these relationships fit with an important issue raised by both Mullender and Ward, and Biegel, that is, that empowerment strategies should exploit the naturally occurring social systems and meeting places.

The importance of ethics

The importance of the ethics of empowerment rests in the need to establish a credible form of practice. For if such practice is to avoid the 'social aerosol' criticism levelled by Mullender and Ward (where the reference is to masking the real situation), then it is important that the value base for practice is subject to a continuous process of evaluation. This evaluation also has to consider and identify the costs and benefits to the person or group. This involves a careful consideration of a number of inter-connected, complementary, but often contradictory outcomes which can be taking place on different levels, psychological, inter-personal, and political. Drawing upon the work of Warwick and Kelman (1976), Fawcett *et al.* (1984) propose the following four-dimensional framework as essential to the evaluation process:

1 The choice of empowerment goals.
2 The selection of targets for empowerment.
3 The choice of means to achieve empowerment.
4 The analysis of the consequences of empowerment for the targets, the change agents and society in general.

The choice of goals

Fawcett *et al.* argue that the choice of goals requires careful consideration, as it is possible that these may be in conflict. Alternatively, they might have both positive and negative aspects. Also, as Mullender and Ward point out, it is important that the individual or group seeking empowerment are totally involved in the process of goal identification and setting. With regard to Margaret, the goals of empowerment must be compatible with her development towards 'participatory competence'. Here the stages identified by Kieffer provide a guide. At first the goals may be solely concerned with the development of a positive self-image and Margaret's establishment within a peer group. This provides the possibility for Margaret to practise early participative skills in a supportive environment. The danger is that goals that are too adventurous, or that are practised in a hostile environment, may bring frustration and failure at this early stage. The consequences of such an over-exposure could be very damaging to the emerging self-definition and self-esteem, with the result that earlier feelings of helplessness are compounded.

The selection of targets

Here it should be noted that while real possibilities exist for the enhancement of self-esteem, there is also the possibility that empowerment may disrupt social harmony. This may result in a reduction in the level and extent of external support that the target(s) receives or is offered. This highlights the negative and positive aspects of the dynamic process of empowerment. For Margaret, becoming a target for empowerment may alter her relationship with John and her father. On the one hand this may lead to personal growth, while on the other hand the relationships may alter to a point where they break down. This process of break-down may be very painful and produce intense feelings of loss.

Moreover, Margaret may lose the positive aspects of these relationships which may be emotional or material. For example, her relationship with her father may break down and she may be forced to leave home. Alternative accommodation may not be as comfort-able, it may be more expensive, or if it is shared it may afford less privacy than before. On the other hand it may force an important step in the direction of independence. This possibility of disruption of social harmony also extends to the centre, where Margaret's movement towards empowerment may be met by resentment from staff members who gained their own self-esteem from a caring but paternalistic relationship with her. In response to Margaret's growing 'participatory competence', obstacles to her progress may be introduced, for example, with the removal of particular supports or even direct discrimination.

The choice of means

Here, Warwick and Kelman propose five broad alternatives: facili-tation, environmental manipulation, persuasion, psychic manipula-tion and coercion. 'Facilitation' involves the removal of obstacles to action, therefore making it easier for individuals or groups to effect their choices. Here changes in the structure of the 'life planning process' may facilitate a situation where individuals can effectively represent their needs as they see them, rather than, as in Margaret's case, where her perception of her needs was ignored, and a different professional perception of need imposed.

On the other hand 'environmental manipulation' involves a deliberate act of changing the structure of alternatives in the environment, for example, by improving leadership skills. For Margaret this could involve assertiveness skills or presentation skills, which would enable her to communicate more effectively. If she becomes very tense and anxious when giving her view then relaxation and other stress management techniques may be effective. These strategies fit with the definition of social technologies referred to above.

'Persuasion' relates to the attempt to change attitudes or the behaviour of others by argument, for example, by demonstrating the consequences. In Margaret's case this might mean the re-negotiation of the relationships that exist between herself and her father, John, and/or the centre, the effect being that these relationships could support the development of 'participatory competence' rather than compounding feelings of helplessness. However, 'psychic manipulation' raises different issues, as this relates to changing personal qualities that effect choice without the knowledge of the person concerned. Fawcett *et al.* argue that:

> This issue might be raised with virtually all empowerment efforts: to what extent are the targets of empowerment efforts aware that their control over their lives will be affected? As effectiveness of empowerment efforts is increased, issues regarding the informed consent of targets of empowerment efforts should assume greater importance.
>
> (Fawcett *et al.* 1984: 155)

This, in contrast with Kieffer, raises the possibility that the empowerment process can begin before a 'sense of personal violation' occurs. Here people may be engaged in a process whereby they came to recognise their oppression. This might be compatible with Freire's concept of 'praxis', referred to earlier.

'Coercion' takes the idea of means one stage further as this seeks to legitimise the use of force when social values are threatened. In the case study it might be seen as coercion if the following circumstances applied: the contracts of workers at the centre contain a section outlining the rights of people using the centre to determine their own wishes, but at the same time it identifies the responsibilities of workers in supporting such choices. This requirement is then reinforced by the threat of disciplinary action if not fulfilled.

The analysis of consequences

Fawcett *et al.* identify this as the critical dimension, as ultimately the ethics of a particular empowerment strategy rest upon the balance of its consequences for the targets, change agent(s) and society. They argue that an ethical strategy must have the targets rather than the change agents as the main beneficiaries of empowerment, and that they should be less rather than more dependent upon professionals. However, they also point out that, in relation to the consequences for society, the integrative values and norms may be destroyed or weakened. From this it can be seen that the potential benefits for Margaret have to be set in a wider context. This has to consider the costs and benefits of the strategy towards empowerment. It is also essential that the change agents or workers are clear as to their motives within this process. This links with Mullender and Ward's insistence that with professional practice that aims to be empowering, the starting point must be to make clear and explicit the value base. It is from this value base that practice must develop.

Managing the paradox

Finally, in the ethical evaluation of empowerment strategies, Fawcett *et al.* conclude by pointing to the complex paradoxical nature of empowerment. First, empowerment is a diverse problem that often requires diverse and apparently contradictory solutions. Second, community empowerment may require individuals to relinquish some degree of personal control or choice. Third, in increasing the capacity for individuals and groups to take control over their own lives, the capacity for the entire community – such as that in the centre Margaret attends – to take one action may be weakened.

CONCLUSION

This chapter has demonstrated the complex nature of the concept of empowerment by identifying its multi-dimensional nature, which includes both psychological and political dimensions. It has pointed out the dangers of using the term 'empowerment' in professional practice without a clear idea of what the concept implies and has therefore sought to clarify the conceptual issues. These ideas were developed through the discussion of a developmental model, and the identification of practical strategies that might facilitate 'participatory competence'.

The case study of Margaret Adams has been used to try to highlight some of the essential elements that need to come together at the beginning of the empowerment process, especially the 'sense of violation' that is essential to the process. The case study also provided a basis for a discussion of the ethical issues. This is important for, as Hess (1984) points out, empowerment is a dynamic process which has both costs and benefits for all those involved.

KEY POINTS

Conflict	Power
Control	Powerlessness
Empowerment	Praxis
Marginalisation	Self-definition
Oppression	Self-determination
Participatory competence	Social technologies
Paternalism	Sociopolitical structures

REFERENCES

Adams, R. (1990) *Self Help, Social Work and Empowerment*, Basingstoke: Macmillan Educational.

Atkinson, D. and Williams, F. (eds) (1990) *Know Me as I am: An Anthology of Prose, Poetry and Art from People with Learning Difficulties*, London: Hodder and Stoughton.

Biegel, D.E. (1984) 'Help seeking and receiving in urban ethnic neighborhoods: strategies for empowerment', *Prevention in Human Services* 3: 119–43.

Brown, C. and Ringma, C. (1989) 'New disability services: the critical role of staff in a consumer directed empowerment model of service for physically disabled people', *Disability, Handicap and Society* 4(3): 241–7.

Crawley, B. (1988) *The Growing Voice*, London: V.I.A.

Fawcett, C.B., Seekins, S., Wang, P.L., Mute, C. and Suarez de Balcazar, Y. (1984) 'Creating and using social technologies for community empowerment', *Prevention in Human Services* 3: 145–71.

Freire, P. (1970) *Pedagogy of the Oppressed*, New York: Seabury Press.

Hess, R. (1984) 'Thoughts on empowerment', *Prevention in Human Services* 3: 227–30.

Hill Collins, P. (1990) *Black Feminist Thought: Knowledge, Consciousness, and the Politics of Empowerment*, London: HarperCollins Academic.

Katz, R. (1984) 'Empowerment and synergy: expanding the community's healing resources', *Prevention in Human Services* 3: 201–26.

Kieffer, C.H. (1984) 'Citizen empowerment: a developmental perspective', *Prevention in Human Services* 3: 9–36.

Loney, M., Bocock, B., Clarke, J., Cochrane, A., Graham, P. and Wilson, M. (1991) *The State or the Market: Politics And Welfare In Contemporary Britain*, London: Sage.

Mullender, A. and Ward, D. (1989) 'Challenging familiar assumptions: preparing for and initiating a self directed group', *Groupwork* 1989 2(1): 5–26.

Mullender, A. and Ward, D. (1991) *Self Directed Groupwork: Users Take Action for Empowerment*, London: Whiting and Birch.

Rappaport, J. (1981) 'In praise of paradox: a social policy of empowerment over prevention', *American Journal Of Community Psychology* 9(1): 1–25.

Rappaport, J. (1984) 'Studies in empowerment: introduction to the issue', *Prevention in Human Services* 3: 1–7.

Rogers, C. (1979) *Carl Rogers on Personal Power*, New York: Delacorte.

Warwick, D.P. and Kelman, H.C. (1976) 'Ethical issues in social intervention', in W.G. Bennis, K.D. Benns, R. Chin and K.E. Corley (eds) *The Planning of Change*, 3rd edn., New York: Holt, Rinehart and Winston.

Part III

Specific interventions

The final part of this book focuses on specific interventions for people with a learning disability. Chapter 6 explores the techniques of behavioural intervention and Chapter 7 examines psychotherapeutic interventions.

When reading these chapters the concepts explored in the earlier parts of the book should be recalled. The issues raised by the ideas of informed choice and empowerment are particularly relevant when examining such interventions. In addition, the chapter on ethical issues will be helpful when considering the ethical dilemmas which frequently occur in the use of specific interventions.

The chapter on behavioural interventions outlines the common behavioural principles, but sets them within the confines of what is considered to be acceptable practice in today's caring services. The emphasis is placed upon valuing people and the use of non-aversive methods for changing behaviour.

The final chapter is also in keeping with modern approaches to care delivery and focuses on what are sometimes termed 'talking cures'. The reasons why people may be considered to require these types of intervention is addressed in the first part of the chapter in relation to the issue of dual diagnosis, that is, where people with a learning disability are also diagnosed as having a behavioural, emotional or mental health problem. These interventions are generally thought of as being client-centred, with the focus on the client–therapist relationship. However, this raises the issue of who has the power within this relationship, as well as who the beneficiaries of the therapy actually are. This clearly links with the concepts outlined in Part I of the book which seeks to answer the questions: for whom services are being provided and whose needs are being met.

Chapter 6

Behavioural approaches

Patricia Brigden and Margaret Todd

INTRODUCTION

The notion that one person should control another person's behaviour is becoming increasingly unacceptable in the 1990s.

In the past, behaviour modification has been linked to social engineering, in recognition of what some saw as its potential to create the sort of scenario described by George Orwell in his book *1984*. This foresaw a world in which people could do nothing without permission and everything they said or did was rewarded or punished according to rigid rules inflexibly applied by Big Brother. By implication, this creates a tragic and unfair situation for individuals whose needs and wishes cannot be met within the established rules. The possibility of such a situation arising has concerned psychologists and others for many years. It is known that behavioural principles can be misapplied, and that clients thereby become victims of abuse. It was pointed out that if you could reward a person for doing more, you could also reward them for doing less, and thus it might be of benefit to some people to teach individuals with a learning disability to sit in the corner and do and say nothing for long periods of time. Thus, even when behaviour modification was at its most influential in the days of institutions, there were those who saw a need for ethical guidelines.

The popularity of different treatment and therapy methods ebbs and flows with social opinion. In the 1960s and 1970s the use of aversive techniques were prominent. These techniques are now considered rarely, if ever, acceptable as treatments in the UK.

As the philosophy of normalisation (Wolfensberger 1972) and ordinary living (King's Fund 1980) has become the dominant philosophy in services for people with a learning disability, it has become totally unacceptable to label or stigmatise people as different. Instead they are to be seen as full members of society, to be treated as anyone would wish to be treated, allbeit with extra support and assistance. It follows that treatment methods must be ones which people offering the treatment would find acceptable for themselves.

People with a learning disability also have citizens' rights. In accordance with this they should have the right to choose how to behave and what treatments they are prepared to accept. Wherever possible they should be consulted, and if it is not possible to directly consult the individual, an advocate or the person who most closely fills this role should be consulted. Sometimes keyworkers and/or family are consulted in lieu of an advocate and this may or may not be good practice. It is, for example, possible that the family's wishes may not be the same as the client's. Likewise keyworkers may unwittingly be representing staff wishes rather than those of their client. Keyworkers may also be very new to their post and/or new to the client in question. This may mean that they have little knowledge about that individual's wishes and needs. To be an advocate a person must know the client very well and must not have a vested interest in the outcome of the decision-making, other than that the decision should be in the best interest of the client and should accord with the client's wishes and needs. A life-planning or individual programme-planning system may be of help in ensuring that client consultation occurs.

As hospitals close and people move into the community into ordinary houses in ordinary streets (King's Fund 1985), both service users and staff start viewing situations differently. Behaviours which may have been tolerated in larger residential settings are no longer acceptable in the smaller dwellings in ordinary streets. In view of this, behavioural techniques continue to be considered as appropriate intervention strategies for some individuals. A variety of behavioural intervention strategies is explored in this chapter. The theory of classical conditioning is explained first, as it forms the basis of all other behavioural techniques described.

CLASSICAL CONDITIONING

'Classical conditioning' or 'Pavlovian conditioning' was first described by the Russian physiologist Ivan Pavlov (1849–1936) from observations of experiments with dogs. The response described are automatic nervous system responses, and as such are not under direct control of the animal.

Pavlov discovered that if he presented a dog with meat (unconditioned stimulus) the dog salivated (unconditioned response). He then rang a bell (conditioned stimulus) each time the dog was presented with meat, and the dog salivated. Eventually the bell was rung without the meat being presented, and the dog would salivate to the sound of the bell (conditioned response). (This concept is represented diagrammatically in Figure 6.1.) In other words, the dog has learned to associate the bell with the presentation of the meat and therefore salivates to the sound of the bell. This kind of learning is thought to explain some learned fear response and phobias.

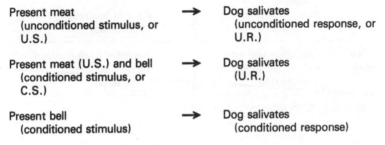

Figure 6.1 Classical conditioning

Classical conditioning is considered to be a law of behaviour. However this is not very useful in practical situations, due to the fact that the responses are not under the direct control of the individual. A behavioural technique which is considered more useful in practical situations is that of operant conditioning.

OPERANT CONDITIONING

Operant conditioning means that the behaviour is affected by its consequences. Four consequences to behaviour are possible.

A behaviour can be followed by:

- a positive or rewarding event, that is, something the individual finds pleasing;
- the removal of an aversive event, that is, something the individual finds disagreeable is removed;

- an aversive event, that is, something the person finds unpleasant is introduced;
- the temporary or permanent loss of a positive event.

These situations are respectively called: positive reinforcement, negative reinforcement, punishment and time out.

Positive and negative reinforcement strengthens the behaviour which precedes it. Punishment and time out both serve to decrease the behaviour which precedes it. This is shown diagrammatically in Figure 6.2.

	Positive	*Negative*
Add	Positive reinforcement/ reward	Punishment
	Rate of behaviour increases ↑	Rate of behaviour decreases ↓
Take away	Extinction and time out Rate of behaviour decreases ↓	Negative reinforcement Rate of behaviour increases ↑

Figure 6.2   Consequences of behaviour

A number of points need to be made about this. First, a reward is something a person will work to achieve and a punishment is something a person will work to avoid. It may be possible to ask people what they find rewarding and what they find punishing. Where this is not possible, it is usual to observe a person's behaviour over a period of time, and from this it is possible to infer which things are experienced as positive and which things are experienced as negative. If this is not done, it is possible that mistaken assumptions can be made about what is experienced as positive or negative. For example, people who enjoy making others angry will be rewarded by the display of verbal and non-verbal signs of anger. People who like to spend time on their own will be pleased to be sent to a room on their own. Thus what was meant to be time out can be experienced by the individual as something rewarding. These effects of behavioural programmes may be interpreted by those implementing them as a failure of the programme. In fact the laws of operant conditions (Figure 6.2) are working well, but programme implementers have failed to understand exactly what is happening.

The four aspects of operant conditioning — positive reinforcement, negative reinforcement, punishment, extinction/time out — are 'natural laws'. They occur constantly in our daily lives and form the main system of social control such as receiving payment (positive reinforcement) in return for work. To observe behaviour in its environmental context and analyse accurately what is going on, it is necessary to understand that much of our behaviour is controlled by negative reinforcement and punishment (as well as by positive reinforcement and extinction/time out). However, for reasons which will be explored, neither is used for treatment and training purposes.

Negative reinforcement, which is defined as removal of an aversive event thereby increasing the rate of behaviour preceding it, is too complex to facilitate easy understanding, an important consideration when devising behavioural programmes. It does however occur in society, for example, with the mother who finds that her baby stops crying when she picks it up. In this case the crying was experienced as aversive by the mother, and the fact that the crying stopped each time the baby was picked up resulted in the mother picking up the baby more often. It is therefore important to recognise from observations such as behavioural situations when this type of dynamic is occurring.

Punishment is defined as administering something unpleasant so as to decrease the behaviour preceding it. This procedure is not recommended for treatment and training purposes: first, because it does not teach a person what to do; second, because it gives the person attention for behaving in a way which is not acceptable and so may actually reward the undesired behaviour; and third, because it loses its effectiveness. As a consequence the punishment becomes increasingly severe to maintain its initial effect. Even if the level of punishment used initially was within reasonable bounds, it will not be in the end. The issue of reasonable bounds is also debatable. That is, what level of punishment is to be considered acceptable for what type of inappropriate behaviour, and to whom is it considered acceptable. It is doubtful whether the person receiving the punishment considers any level of punishment acceptable.

The dangers of using physical punishment are that it would increase in intensity and frequency until a level of physical abuse was reached. It would also be difficult to control the various different people who would be administering the punishment. For these reasons:

- it is helpful to have staff guidelines that expressly forbid this kind of treatment;
- if staff are forbidden to use certain treatment methods it is helpful to give them advice on what is considered a more acceptable alternative;
- before doing so it is worth considering the reasons for wishing to decrease the behaviours.

An individual's behaviour may have several unwanted effects. It may disrupt the lives of those people who share the living environment or the working environment. It may also interfere with the learning of new skills. In addition, it may mean that others do not want to spend time with the individual. This may be because people who try to do so feel punished by the negative outcome of the interaction and so feel less inclined to try again. Finally, the behaviour may cause real damage to the person concerned and to others. Self-damage, such as severe head banging, can be severe enough to be life threatening.

DECREASING BEHAVIOURS

Recommended methods of decreasing behaviour may be summarised as:

- ensuring reinforcement of good behaviours;
- teaching incompatible skill(s);
- taking away something pleasant, as in extinction, time out and response costs, and, in certain circumstances, over-correction or a form of minimalised 'restraint'.

These techniques need definition to ensure clarity.

Ensuring reinforcement of good behaviour

Carers tend to breathe a sigh of relief when the people they care for are quiet, as this provides them with a chance to get on with other things. Giving people attention when they are behaving appropriately is likely to increase the appropriate behaviour. Equally people should receive minimal attention when they are behaving in unacceptable ways, thus reducing the likelihood of this behaviour occurring in the future.

One of the rules used to justify the existence of programmes for decreasing behaviour in the 1990s is that there must be clear evidence that every effort has been made in a consistent and documented manner to implement reinforcement of good behaviour. Even when this has failed to work on its own, it should be seen to be occurring in conjunction with other behavioural change methods. Progress should be evaluated and kept under review.

Teaching an incompatible skill

The rationale for this approach is that some skills cannot be performed simultaneously. Teaching positive skills that cannot be carried out at the same time as the unwanted behaviours will eventually replace the negative behaviour. However, it is important to identify the right skill to teach. The individual must want to learn this skill and must gain a measure of pleasure from it which is greater than that which they receive from the unwanted behaviour.

Long periods of time with little to keep oneself occupied is well known to trigger inventive ways of filling time. Prisoners and hostages have reported using stones to scratch a calendar on the wall, or making a game of noughts and crosses on the floor. They have also been inventive about using heating pipes for communicating with others.

These are examples of inventive ways to use time, given little or no resources. Unfortunately some people with a learning disability use anti-social methods of filling time. To prevent this happening every effort should be made to fill time with constructive activity (this may develop the incompatible skills), thereby channelling people's behaviour in a more healthy productive fashion. While people are constructively occupied, they do not have time to carry out anti-social or undesirable behaviours. This strategy will reduce or eliminate these behaviours, and will also prevent the unwanted behaviours from developing in the first place. There is already much evidence that school leavers with a learning disability do not display the range and severity of behaviours that were common in the institutions in the past. In relation to these school leavers, adult services have a responsibility to at least maintain and preferably improve their level of constructive skills which will compete with undesired behaviours.

Taking away something pleasant

Extinction

Extinction means the withdrawal of reinforcements from previously reinforced behaviours. For example, if a person usually receives a reward following a behaviour, but then gradually finds that this behaviour no longer results in the reward, then the person becomes less likely to do the same thing again when next in that situation.

Caution is necessary when considering using this method. The unwanted behaviour usually increases in duration or frequency before improvement occurs. This issue of the behaviour deteriorating before improvement occurs means that this is a dangerous technique to use with people who exhibit self-injurious behaviour. If there is a danger of making them worse it may be considered unethical and maybe life-threatening. Prior to using extinction programmes, all those concerned need to reassure themselves that they will be able to tolerate the exacerbation of the behaviour, and see it through to the point where the individual with a learning disability eventually realises that the behaviour is not going to be rewarded by attention, and eventually stops carrying out this behaviour.

However, if a behavioural programme addresses the issue of decreasing undesirable behaviours without considering positive alternatives to replace these behaviours, then other undesirable behaviours may occur to replace them. As previously stated, people find inventive ways to fill unoccupied time.

Time out

Time out involves transferring an individual from a more reinforcing to a less reinforcing situation following a particular behaviour (Van Houten *et al.* 1988). This does not necessarily mean physically removing the individual from the environment but it does mean removing reinforcement from the individual. The various types of reinforcement will be considered.

Time out may involve exclusion. Exclusionary time out consists of removing the person from the situation in which reinforcement is occurring for a short period of time such as five minutes. This should be done in the least drastic manner available. Thus it might be sufficient to leave the living room and stay in the hall or kitchen for up to five minutes, or it might be enough to stand beyond a room partition for a count of twenty, for example. Although a special room (time out room) may be used, this is often unnecessary. A room used for this purpose needs to be bare of reinforcers. This is one reason why a bedroom may not be an acceptable place to use. A second reason why a bedroom may not be acceptable is that it may not be within easy reach for the staff.

It is important that the period used for time out is never more than ten to fifteen minutes (DHSS 1983). While a person is in exclusionary time out, staff should be observing the individual. Staff should not wait for a time period to elapse, but as soon as the person is quiet they should be asked if they are ready to resume the activity. If the person acquiesces they should then return to the activity. If they do not become calm then a little longer should be allowed. However the period must not exceed ten to fifteen minutes as this situation then becomes seclusion and within a behavioural programme this is classed as a punishment and thereby an unacceptable practice. If the period of time out has to be restarted more than once because the person remains disruptive, angry and aggressive, it is likely the person has become genuinely upset and needs comforting. If this approach does not help, and the problem continues, this could be an indication that a multi-disciplinary case conference is needed to explore further what is happening and whether the best approach is being used.

Time out need not be exclusionary in nature. Non-exclusionary time out consists of introducing into the situation a stimulus associated with less reinforcement (Foxx and Shapiro 1978).

Partial time out is also possible. Examples include turning one's back on the person for a count of ten (where interaction and reading the facial expression are the reinforcers), turning the television or radio off for ten seconds, removing an item such as a book or toy for ten seconds. It may also be enough to move a person to a table on their own on the edge of the dining room when they are disruptive at meal times. This is a less drastic reaction than taking the person away to a time out room.

If time out is used, some rules and guidelines are essential. The least drastic method is always the method of preference. Thus partial time out is preferable to exclusionary time out. Time out should not be used at all if a positive programme can be used instead, and a positive programme should always be used in conjunction with time out. In order to maintain good practice the following guidelines are recommended:

1 Advice from a qualified therapist or psychologist should be sought prior to utilising time out.
2 The time out procedure to be followed should be included in the individual's care plan/programme plan. This plan should be supervised by a qualified therapist or psychologist.
3 Partial time out should be used in the first instance, prior to any other form of time out being utilised.
4 All forms of time out should be recorded and monitored.
5 Time out should never last longer than fifteen minutes.
6 Staff should request service guidelines on the use of time out.

Time out is not a behavioural method to use without due consideration, or to be complacent about, nor should it be assumed that one is a competent practitioner and can therefore manage without expert advice. It is good practice to record the thinking process the group went through in deciding the type of time out or the time out location, as this can be used to justify the claim that the least drastic method was used.

Response cost

This involves removing an amount of reinforcer following a particular behaviour, for example, library fines and parking tickets. It can be used in programmes where clients earn tokens.

Over-correction

An example of this would be setting right the environment that has been disturbed or disrupted by the undesirable behaviour, but over-doing the correction. Over-correction is a punishment which has no advantages over other punishment methods except that it may be more socially acceptable than other forms of punishment (Webster and Azrin 1973). It is subject to the same ethical considerations as other punishment procedures.

Restraint

This is generally an unacceptable procedure to be included in a behavioural programme. A minimalised form of restraint may be useful. For example, if a person habitually grabs food at meal times it can be effective to hold down the hand while counting to ten each time the person attempts to grab the food.

Ascertaining the reasons for the behaviour

Difficulties with client behaviour usually start with vague, poorly defined complaints about disruptive behaviour. These poorly defined complaints are sometimes described as 'fuzzies'. That is, they can be interpreted differently by different people. Disruptive behaviour may mean screaming and shouting or hair-pulling or hitting others and so on. The first step is to try to clarify what it is that is being complained about. It is helpful to be able to define the behaviour in performance statements such as 'pulls other people's hair' (Open University Course Team 1982). Staff need to think through what the problem is until as a group they agree on a performance statement of what the issue is. Once the behaviour can be clearly stated, it is necessary to consider what the antecedents are, that is, what is happening just before the incident occurs. The antecedents may be the trigger to the behaviour. Details of the background to incidents are important, as there is often a pattern to events. It is possible that the behaviour is under the control of the antecedents and any behavioural strategy will need to address this issue. In these cases, it is possible that if the antecedents are eliminated, the behaviours will not occur.

It is also important to identify the consequences of the behaviour, as the behaviour may be under the control of what happens after the behaviour occurs. In this instance changing the consequences of the behaviour may eliminate the behaviours.

Recording incidents of behaviours, with details of their antecedents and consequences, is called ABC charting (*a*ntecedents, *b*ehaviour, *c*onsequences) and ABC charts are readily available (see Figure 6.3). After a period of time, depending on the frequency of incidents, and therefore how quickly data can be assembled, consideration is given to what is happening and whether anything can be done to make the behaviour less likely to occur in the future, either by changing the antecedents or the consequences.

Self-injurious behaviour – a recommended approach

Treatments for self-injury tend to be utilised in the following order. First, restraint and/or protective clothing is often used, for example, mittens to prevent hand biting, a helmet to prevent head banging. The least restrictive appliance compatible with response prevention should always be the choice. Second, drugs are often prescribed.

Antecedent Behaviour Consequences Recording Chart

Name ....

Date ....

The Problem
Describe what s/he actually did during the incident.
How long did the behaviour last?
Staff members involved?

Antecedents
What was s/he doing prior to the incident?
What were the first signs?
What actually immediately preceded the incident (e.g. what was
  s/he asked to do etc.)?

Background
Where and at what time did the incident take place?
Who else was involved (non-staff)?

Consequences
How did the incident come to an end?
What did the members of staff do after the incident?
What was happening ten minutes later?

Figure 6.3   ABC chart

Use of medication for this purpose is controversial, and a positive
outcome is largely unproven. There are, however, those who think
there may be future potential in the use of chemotherapy to treat
self-injurious behaviour. According to Schroeder *et al.* (1985), 32
per cent of people who exhibit self-injurious behaviour can be
helped using drugs. Drugs can also be combined with behavioural
techniques. The third option is the use of behavioural treatments,
of which a wide range of techniques are available. Schroeder *et al.*
(1985) found that 94 per cent of people who inflict self-injury were
helped using behavioural treatments. While there are psycho-
dynamic explanations of self-injurious behaviour, there are as yet
no suitable psychoanalytical/psychotherapeutic treatments. The
recommended approach to a client manifesting self-injurious behaviour is to carry out ABC charting, and to obtain a precise description or performance statement of the form the self-injury takes.

The following are examples of the antecedents, behaviour, and consequences in people with self-injurious behaviour.

Antecedent	→	Behaviour	→	Consequences
staff want Fred to wash his clothing		self-injurious behaviour		Fred allowed not to do the clothes washing

In this situation, the recommended treatment would be the behavioural approach.

Antecedent	→	Behaviour	→	Consequences
earache		self-injurious behaviour		medical diagnosis

In this situation, the recommended treatment would be antibiotics and pain killers.

From the second example it can be seen that it is important to ensure that there is not a medical cause for the self-injurious behaviour. If the behaviour is caused by a medical condition then the condition should be treated by the appropriate medical intervention.

It is also important to ensure that staff are not unintentionally reinforcing self-injurious behaviour. This can happen in various ways, including providing desired attention at the wrong times.

For many people, self-injurious behaviour is a form of self-stimulation. Blind people often poke, punch and pull for a feeling sensation. If self-injury is a form of self-stimulation, then it helps to replace the behaviour with a more acceptable form of stimulation such as vibration, touch and sound.

It is important to ensure that tender loving care is never contingent on self-injury. This often happens when desperate parents and/or carers feel sorry for their loved one and perhaps feel they may be behaving in this way because they are unhappy. These feelings can lead to guilt and this can lead to tender loving care being provided only when the person has been inflicting self-injury.

Positive reinforcement alone has not been found to be very effective with self-injurious behaviour. It needs to be combined with other procedures. Thus staff can positively reinforce all types of non-self-injurious behaviour, or positively reinforce behaviours which are incompatible with self-injury.

Relaxation is a useful incompatible behaviour. If a person is injuring themselves using their hands, it is possible to teach them to relax first one hand and then the other. Systematic desensitisation, that is, gradually exposing a person to feared situations and/or stimuli, can be used to help people cope with change, for example, to reduce and stop the wearing of restraints.

If one ceases to reinforce self-injurious behaviour it will eventually disappear (extinction). However, as has already been stated, the behaviour can be expected to deteriorate initially. This means that extinction is likely to be not only unethical, but could be dangerous, and even on occasion life-threatening.

If positive reinforcement and differential reinforcement of other behaviour, relaxation and desensitisation have not worked, then time out or over-correction are possible options. However, advice should be sought before using these techniques. If used, these methods should always be combined with reinforcement of non-self-injurious behaviour.

Combined treatments are more successful than treatments used individually. Thus if restraints are to be phased out as part of a behavioural programme, the client should be taught self-control simultaneously. The anti-psychotic drug Haloperidol, plus behavioural treatment, is often more effective than either treatment alone.

Self-injurious behaviour often reappears following a successful treatment programme. In view of this it may be necessary to change one's approach at regular intervals. This is because the novelty of an approach appears to have the best effect (Murphy and Wilson 1985).

Decreasing behaviours: summary

When decreasing behaviours, the best approach is prevention or developing incompatible behaviours. The more positive skills people have, and the more opportunities they have to put them into practice, and to learn new and better ways of doing things, the less negative behaviour there will be.

When considering adopting a positive approach, staff and carers should be aware of their own usual approach. The 'soft' person gives in to anything for a quiet life while the 'hard' person always has better things to do. The positive person takes the initiative. Staff who want to make residents happy, which in turn makes staff happy, have to become positive people. People are born but relationships are made. Staff are the main people who can make a residence or group home a happy or unhappy place. How things turn out will depend on how residents are treated by staff.

Most parents/carers/staff are a mixture of the types described because they are human. However, anyone can become positive in approach for more of the time. To adopt a positive approach it is necesary to have a clear idea of what the desired outcome will be. It is important to have clear goals, for example, you want the person to behave in a socially acceptable manner in the community. The approach taken must be used consistently, that is, the person must be treated in the same way, every time they do the same thing.

The first and most important method used to increase behaviours is the use of positive reinforcers.

INCREASING BEHAVIOURS

Positive reinforcers

If behaviour is followed by a positive reinforcer it is more likely to happen again. The positive carer always rewards a person for all attempts at the desired behaviour. Reinforcers are used to indicate to the person that he or she is succeeding, that succeeding is fun, and that carers and others are pleased by this success.

A positive reinforcer is defined as something a person is prepared to work for at one particular time. Thus a person might do anything for a cup of coffee first thing in the morning, but will be far less interested if they have just had a cup of coffee and are therefore temporarily satiated. Positive reinforcers fit into four categories:

1 Primary – these are automatically reinforcing items such as food.
2 Secondary – these are items like money and tokens, which are not automatically reinforcing but come to be associated with rewards over time.
3 Social – praise, hugs, kisses and smiles.
4 Stimulation – these can be sensory or tactile, vibration, texture, sound, smell, light.

Social rewards, especially praise and smiles, are very powerful and are often the first choice. However, they are not usually strong enough when used alone and in the first instance they need to be used with other reinforcers. The other reinforcers should be gradually phased out, and the person will have learned or relearned to respond appropriately to social rewards.

When social rewards are not strong enough alone it is useful to try activities. An activity is something a person likes to do. The Premack Principle is an important concept to consider at this point. The Premack Principle relates to positively reinforcing behaviour. It operates when the preferred activity follows a less preferred activity, that is, the person knows that when they have done an activity they dislike they will then be able to do an activity of their choice or something they like. If activities do not work as reinforcers, then primary or secondary reinforcers should be used. However, it is important to ascertain what the person likes best and use these as the reinforcers. The important concept is that reinforcers are the individual's choice. It should never be assumed that what is reinforcing for one person will also be reinforcing for another. Where possible individuals should be asked what their preferences are and should be consulted throughout on the need for any behavioural programme. Drawing up a formal signed contract is excellent practice.

Where an individual is unable to communicate his or her choice, it may be necessary to observe them closely for a number of weeks prior to implementing a behavioural programme. Individuals can be observed in their normal living environment to ascertain what their preferred way of spending time is. They can be observed to ascertain what drinks and foodstuffs they prefer. It is a good idea to introduce the same person to new activities and experiences as these could become reinforcers.

Sensory stimulation can be an important source of reinforcers for people with profound learning disabilities and multiple disabilities including sensory disabilities.

Giving reinforcers

There are five rules in relation to giving reinforcers:

1 Reinforce the person as soon as they do what you want them to do.
2 At first, reward every time the person attempts to do what you want.

3 Reward less often as the individual finds it easier to do something.
4 Always praise the individual even when using other types of reinforcers.
5 Always say exactly why you are pleased with them.

Schedules of reinforcement

Reinforcement schedules represent various ways of reducing the number of times a person is reinforced for the target behaviour without it becoming so infrequent that it is in danger of becoming 'extinction'.

Just as people playing a fruit machine keep playing because they know that occasionally they win the jackpot, so individuals with a learning disability will continue with the target behaviour because they are sure that on occasion they will be reinforced.

The various kinds of reinforcement schedule are shown in Figure 6.4. Reinforcement schedules may be continuous or intermittent. A continuous schedule is where reinforcement follows every appropriate response. This schedule of reinforcement should be used when first trying to establish a behaviour. An intermittent schedule is introduced once the behaviour is established, and is designed to maintain the behaviour. It involves reinforcement following certain responses only.

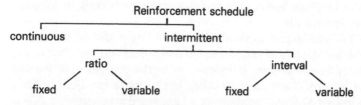

Figure 6.4 Reinforcement schedules

An intermittent schedule may be either a ratio or interval schedule. A ratio schedule depends on the frequency of appropriate responses, that is, the person receives reinforcement for every second or third performance of the behaviour. An interval schedule depends on a response following a specified lapse of time, that is, the person is reinforced after every fifteen or thirty seconds that he or she is participating in an activity. Both ratio and interval schedules can be either fixed or variable. Fixed schedules involve giving reinforcement regularly, either after a specified number of responses or after a specified time scale. Variable schedules involve reinforcements following after numbers of responses or periods of time, that can vary but which average out at certain specified numbers or times. An example of a variable schedule is shown below.

Responses									
Reinforcement	**	*	*	*	*	*	*	*	*
Response no.	12	6	8	13	19	24	29	30	32
No. of responses intervening	11	4	2	5	6	5	1	1	2

With reinforcement given ten times for a total of thirty-two responses the average number of responses per reinforcement is three, though the actual number varies considerably.

Reinforcement schedules have advantages and disadvantages. The advantages of continuous schedules are that they are effective for establishing new behaviour and they are easy to administer within structured sessions. The disadvantages of continuous schedules are that they do not reflect real life and they are less resistant to extinction.

The advantages of intermittent schedules are that they are nearer to real life and they are more resistant to extinction. The disadvantages of intermittent schedules are that they are less effective for establishing new behaviours and they are more difficult to administer systematically.

While the jargon used may be off-putting it should be remembered that the aim of reinforcement schedules is simple. That is, the level of reinforcement is reduced once the response pattern has been learned. Care must be taken not to move too quickly from continuous or fixed schedules to a haphazard arrangement. This is because reinforcement can become so infrequent that the behaviour will be extinguished.

Token economy

The token economy is an application of operant conditioning theory that was invented specifically as a treatment for people with learning disabilities who lived in hospitals. Individualised programmes, however, can still usefully form part of an agreed treatment contract between therapist and client. The basic idea is to motivate people to behave more appropriately and constructively by giving them tokens whenever they behave in the predetermined way. The tokens have an incentive function and can be exchanged for a number of different things, such as pleasant single room accommodation, depending on what is agreed and written into the token economy programme.

It is important that the items/events earned are optional extras and not basic rights. It is also important that clients have participated in agreeing that there is a need for such a programme and have willingly agreed to participate in what they perceive is for their own good. The theory of operant conditioning is that not only does the token motivate people to behave in certain ways, but reinforces their behaviours. Such reinforced behaviours should eventually become an integral part of the individual, and will continue even when the token is removed. Figure 6.5 shows an example of individualised token economy programme, discussed and agreed with the client.

Ways of learning new skills

If a person does not know how to perform a certain action, the use of reinforcers is of limited value as the individual will not know which action is being reinforced. In this case the person has to be taught the required action. One method of learning is to copy others. Demonstrating to someone how to do something and encouraging them to imitate the actions can help. When learning a new skill a person should be guided during the difficult stages. It is important to allow people to perform a new skill on their own when they can. Thus, to start with a person might need prompts. Initially, physical prompting, or hand on hand, may be needed. As the individual gains the skill the level of prompting may be reduced to gestural prompts, such as pointing. The level of prompting will be further reduced to verbal prompts, which act as reminders to the individual. Eventually the individual will be able to perform the skill without any prompting.

Task analysis

Task analysis is a process whereby difficult tasks are broken down into small steps. The person is praised every time he or she attempts to perform one step of the skill. As the individual acquires this

	Mon	Tues	Wed	Thur	Fri	Sat	Sun
Self-care completed and bed made by agreed time							
Polite and considerate (no abuse)							
Goes to work experience							
Self-help/household tasks completed							
Rubbish cleared from bedroom							
Bedroom tidy/ clothing put away							

Key: Y = Yes; N = No
Please enter correct code in appropriate column. To be reviewed during one-to-one chat session.

Figure 6.5 Personalised token economy programme

stage he or she is then taught the next stage of the task, and again the person is praised for attempting this step. This process continues until the individual can perform the whole task. Often the task is taught by a process of backward chaining. That is, the last stage of the task is taught first. This provides individuals with a sense of achievement as the task is completed following their effort.

Figure 6.6 is an example of a task analysis for tooth brushing. It can be seen that a scoring method is built in to enable staff to evaluate the levels of prompting needed for the different steps on a weekly basis. This enables staff to decide which steps are being successfully learned and which steps are proving to be difficult.

A second point to note is the need for performance statements, as it may be unclear what some of these instructions mean. A performance statement for the instruction to 'Brush the inside surfaces of the teeth' could be: 'The individual should brush the biting surfaces of the upper and lower teeth on both sides and in the centre of the mouth using a back and forth motion for at least thirty seconds'. Such definitions make it very clear to staff and the client what they are doing and what they are expected to do. Clarity of goals is one key to the success of behavioural interventions.

Tooth brushing

Name ....

Scoring method:
Unco-operative or complete fail	Score 0
Needs complete physical guidance	Score 1
Needs gestural guidance	Score 2
Needs only verbal guidance	Score 3
Performs action completely without prompts	Score 4

Task	Week			
	1	2	3	4
Pick up and hold toothbrush				
Wet the toothbrush				
Remove cap from toothpaste				
Apply toothpaste to brush				
Replace cap on toothpaste				
Brush outside surfaces of teeth				
Brush biting surfaces of teeth				
Brush inside surfaces of teeth				
Fill the cup with water				
Rinse the mouth				
Wipe the mouth				
Rinse the toothbrush				
Put the equipment away				

Figure 6.6   Task analysis and progress chart

What next?

As the environment and social climate continues to change, a number of developments in the application of behavioural technology have occurred. First, there is a great emphasis on ensuring that clients occupy their time constructively. This trend started with ideas such as room management and have become increasingly ambitious as those responsible for service development have become more interested in creating opportunities. As community care continues to develop, integrated activities such as leisure will also develop (Rose 1993).

Second, behavioural principles have become built into systems set up to identify and meet the holistic needs of the person, such as individual programme planning and the constructional approach (Zarkowska and Clements 1988).

The individual programme planning approach involves an endless loop of assessing (to identify needs and long-term goals), planning (to identify short-term goals), implementing (action to meet goals), and evaluating (following up the process), which leads back to assessing and completes the loop. The constructional approach elaborates on the individual programme planning by specifying where and how the behavioural element fits into the framework. It also emphasises the importance of the environment in relation to the client's behaviour. In addition to this, self-management is also a feature of this approach.

With the increasing number of people with learning disabilities living an ordinary life, there is also an increase in the number of individuals with a mild learning disability who have also a range of mental health difficulties. These problems require the same range of treatments as the usual adult mental health client group. The need to develop self-control will become important with some individuals. To enable the client to gain skills in self-control, the therapist must specify the problem with the client, establish a commitment to change and measure the frequency of relevant behaviours. This will involve the therapist in collecting data, analysing causes, and designing a programme to help the client manage the situation, the behaviour and the consequences. It is important to ensure support for the programme from the relevant staff/carer.

A typical contract with a client includes: target behaviours, method of data collection, the reinforcers to be used, the schedule of delivery and who will deliver them, potential problems and their resolutions, bonus and/or penalty clauses, a review date, signatures of all persons involved and the date of the agreement. Once the goal has been attained, consideration needs to be given to maintaining progress over the longer term. Checks can be set up in the form of evaluation strategies, which, in the case of failure result in reintroducing the programme for an agreed period of time. Getting together with someone at regular intervals to check on the progress will greatly assist in making the success last.

Behaviour-changing techniques

Systematic desensitisation

This procedure involves a client being taken through a hierarchy of real or imagined anxiety-producing situations, starting with those eliciting least anxiety, and progressing gradually to those eliciting most anxiety, while being encouraged to remain in a relaxed state. This is well known to be an effective treatment for anxiety states. However, systematic self-desensitisation is now popular. This uses the same process but clients go through the stages by themselves. This is an example of self-modification.

The technique may work, for example, by clients learning to construct their own fear hierarchy, and teaching themselves deep muscle relaxation, possibly utilising tapes and self-teaching programmes. Following this they then work through the therapy steps. Though this may be difficult for a person with a learning disability to do unaided, this clear trend in treatment towards self-management should be noted.

Cognitive behaviour modification

This important development acknowledges the importance of beliefs, thoughts and perceptions, and the need to stop unproductive, debilitating thoughts and beliefs and replace them with positive and constructive ones; so, for example, 'I cannot' becomes 'I can'. The importance of imagery is central to the concept. Behaviour modifiers assist clients to screen their thoughts, private verbal behaviour and/or images and either stop them, replace them or reinterpret them. Thus behaviour modifiers are interested in what goes on inside the person.

Gentle teaching

This represents another facet of changing behaviour. Gentle teaching, a phrase first coined by McGee and colleagues (1987), is based on using non-aversive techniques for dealing with challenging behaviour. Marginalised people need to be especially valued on a non-consequential basis. Behaviours occur for a reason and are sometimes a logical response to the absurdities in the environment in which people find themselves. Bonding, friendship, trust and security are all felt to be important. Person-specific reciprocal relationships need to be made between each individual carer and client. This tends to be seen as holistic, humanistic thinking. It has also been seen as anti-behavioural. On closer examination, however, it relies heavily on functional analysis. ABC charting is one method of conducting a functional analysis and, as stated earlier, this is a behavioural technique. Gentle teaching also relies on environmental/ecological manipulation, which is also a behavioural strategy. Gentle teaching also disagrees with the use of aversive and punishment techniques, and modern behavioural practitioners also now disagree with these techniques. Both are responding to the climate of social opinion that aversive/negative methods are unacceptable.

CASE STUDY – MATT

Matt, aged 24, has a life-long history of aggressive behaviour which has led to his exclusion from several schools. Prior to starting at the day centre there had been a history of episodic aggression at the health service day-care service, and the psychologist had been intensively involved with him. Matt commenced attending the centre on a part-time basis when the special needs base opened. This attendance had been successful for sixteen months. There had been occasional incidents of aggression, such as kicking, but the staff felt confident to deal with these episodes. It was decided to offer him a full-time place at the centre, but this led to a rise in the level of challenging behaviour. Incidents of physical aggression became almost daily occurrences and, although most were managed effectively, on some occasions Matt had to be physically restrained by three members of staff. During one of these incidents a member of staff received a severe bite. Staff injuries escalated in the three months after Matt started full-time attendance. The incidents were usually kicking. The staff resolved this by ensuring that Matt was provided with soft footwear to put on when he entered the centre. However, Matt then commenced to punch staff, which he had not done previously.

The policy of the centre is to try to ensure that clients are not excluded because of aggressive behaviour. Due to the increased level of challenging behaviour it was decided to implement a behavioural programme for Matt.

Matt is known to have brain damage and complex partial epilepsy. Many of the drugs used to control this are contra-indicated because of exceptionally severe side effects experienced by Matt. His abilities are patchy: he is able to read and write and do simple arithmetic at a 6-year-old ability level. His expressive language and overt behaviour are obsessive in nature. Interrupting him in an obsessive-compulsive sequence results in violent behaviour such as kicking, biting and hitting, but much of the violence can be avoided, especially in recurrent behaviours. For example, Matt has repeatedly refused to come out of a cupboard where he throws things at the electric meters, threatening his own safety and making it likely that the electricity supply will be fused. He can be diverted from this activity by asking him to lock the door and to replace the key in the office.

Matt's behaviour varies according to whether epileptic seizures are imminent, so it is presumably due to temporal lobe auras. Staff must therefore be able to perceive these warnings and adapt their behaviours accordingly. When Matt is in a co-operative mood he will join in activities willingly, provided they are ones in which he is interested and enjoys. However, if his behaviour is of an obsessive-compulsive nature he should be allowed to set the pace for the day's activities. A flexible routine and constant empathic handling are crucial.

Suggested approach

First it is important to establish clearly in performance terms what it is that staff are concerned about. It is then necessary to complete ABC charting to ascertain the frequency and severity of incidents actually occurring as well as ascertaining the function of the behaviour.

As Matt has a pattern of aggressive behaviour it is worth considering the types of skills or activities that could be developed or used to prevent the aggression from occurring. This raises the issue of how Matt spends his time, and whether this could be constructed so that Matt was purposefully occupied for much of his time.

Reinforcers need to be identified for Matt and used to develop competing constructive behaviours. It would be difficult to use exclusionary time out because Matt cannot be physically moved at the times when this might be warranted. In addition to this Matt enjoys being on his own, therefore removing him from the room after a violent episode has occurred is likely to be reinforcing for Matt, thus making the behaviour more likely to occur in the future. However, encouraging Matt to go to a quiet area voluntarily when he gets angry would help to avoid potential incidents.

Extinction might be dangerous to implement due to the fact that the behaviour tends to deteriorate before it improves. Indeed staff ignoring incidents may be one reason why Matt's behaviour has deteriorated in recent months, for example, when kicking people didn't work he started to thump them instead in a continued effort to gain attention. Matt might well have learned that escalating violence is a method of gaining attention.

The attitude of staff was relevant to Matt's treatment programme. Staff adopted a more positive approach and became more
consistent in their treatment of him. The individual programme
plan and/or constructional approach are both useful in working
with Matt, to assist in helping to maintain the creation of opportunities for using time constructively under regular review.

KEY POINTS

Antecedents	Over-correction
Aversive techniques	Positive reinforcement
Classical conditioning	Prompting
Consequences	Response cost
Extinction	Restraint
Incompatible skills	Self-injurious behaviour
Negative reinforcement	Task analysis
Non-aversive techniques	Time out
Operant conditioning	

REFERENCES

Department of Health (DoH) (1991) *The National Health Service and
    Community Care Act*, London: HMSO.
DoH (1993) *The Mental Health Act Section 118, Draft Code of Conduct*,
    London: HMSO.
Department of Health and Social Security (DHSS) (1983) *Mental Health
    Act*, London: HMSO.
Foxx, R. and Shapiro, S. (1978) 'The time out ribbon: A non-exclusionary
    time out procedure', *Journal of Applied Behavioural Analysis* 11:
    125–36.
King's Fund (1985) *An Ordinary Life*, London: King's Fund Centre.
McGee, J., Menolascino, F., Hobbs, D. and Menousek, P. (1987) *Gentle
    Teaching: A Non-Aversive Approach to Helping Persons with Mental
    Retardation*, New York: Human Sciences Press Inc.
Martin, G. and Pear, J. (1992) *Behaviour Modification: What Is It and
    How To Do It*, New York: Simon and Schuster.
Murphy, G. and Wilson, B. (1985) *Self-injurious Behaviour*, Kidder-
    minster: BIMH.
Open University Course Team (1982) *The Handicapped Person in the
    Community, Block 2 Unit 5*, Milton Keynes: Open University Press.
Rose, S. (1993) 'Integrated leisure activities' in P. Brigden and M. Todd
    (eds), *Concepts in Community Care for People with a Learning Diffi-
    culty*, Basingstoke: Macmillan.
Schroeder, S., Schroeder, C., Smith, B. and Dolldorf, J. (1985) 'Preva-
    lence in self injurious behaviour in a large state facility for the retarded: a

three year follow up study' in G. Murphy and B. Wilson (eds), *Self Injurious Behaviour*, Kidderminster: BIMH.

Van Houten, R., Axelrod, S., Bailey, J., Favell, J., Foxx, R., Iwota, B. and Louass, O. (1988) 'The right to effective behavioural treatments', *Journal of Applied Behavioural Analysis* 21(4): 381–4.

Webster, D. and Azrin, N. (1973) 'Required relaxation: A method of inhibiting agitative-disruptive behaviour of retardates', *Behaviour Research and Therapy* 11: 67–78.

Wolfensberger, W. (1972) *The Principles of Normalisation in Human Services*, Toronto: National Institute on Mental Retardation.

Zarkowska, E. and Clements, J. (1988) *Challenging Behaviour: the Constructional Approach*, London: Chapman and Hall.

Chapter 7

Psychotherapeutic interventions

Julia Lloyd and Margaret Todd

INTRODUCTION

One result of the philosophical ideal of normalisation (Wolfensberger 1972) has been commitment to the idea that people with learning disabilities who also have behavioural, emotional or psychiatric problems should continue to receive care in the community, so long as they are not at risk. There may be difficulties in achieving this goal for such dually diagnosed people, but a practical result has been greater accessibility for them to the wider range of therapeutic processes available in the community. According to the principles of normalisation, people with learning disabilities have the right to the same treatment as those without a handicap (Skene 1991).

Some studies point to a greater prevalence of disturbed behaviour in institutions than in the community (Mulick and Kedesdy 1988), as one effect of institutionalisation is an increase in psychiatric problems. But community care programmes, where people with a learning disability are discharged from institutions to ordinary houses, are making deviant behaviour more visible in society, even though clients with severe behavioural problems may be less likely to be selected for community placement. A more normal environment does not necessarily result in client normalisation. On the other hand, people with a learning disability may not experience additional behavioural, emotional or mental health problems, as these problems do not necessarily occur as a result of a learning disability. In fact, mental illness is not a natural concomitant of learning disability (Menolascino and Stark 1984). There are disagreements about the incidence of people with a learning disability with these additional difficulties. Consequently, the first section of this chapter explores the issues arising from the concept of dual diagnosis.

At the same time, it has been stated that individuals with a learning disability are as likely, or more likely than non-learning disabled people to have mental health difficulties (Menolascino and Stark 1984). Thus a range of psychotherapeutic interventions may be required to meet the needs of such individuals. The second section of this chapter therefore briefly outlines the main kinds of psychotherapeutic intervention available and identifies the beliefs held about the nature of the individual from each perspective. The final section presents two case studies to enable the reader to understand the complexities associated with the use of psychotherapeutic interventions with people with a learning disability.

PEOPLE WITH A DUAL DIAGNOSIS

The data yielded on the rates of dual diagnosis has been conflicting, owing to a lack of methodological consistency. Definitions of particular problems and the method of diagnosis have varied across studies. This is compounded by the difficulties of diagnosis of mental health conditions in people with severe learning disabilities (Reid 1982). Estimates of the rate of dual diagnosis range from 15–25 per cent (Jacobsen 1982, Menolascino and Stark 1984, Szymanski and Tanguay 1986). Problems and difficulties often occur simply because people with learning disabilities are treated as a race apart, and so their needs often go unmet during critical periods of their lives because normal support networks are not available. People who are incapable of expressing themselves verbally may be treated as if they have no feelings. Their restricted social circle means that they are deprived of normal social help in times of crises, which may be handled by removing the person from the presented situation instead of looking for other solutions. This causes a far greater degree of disruption to these people's lives than would have occurred if they were receiving the normal types of support. In childhood they may have encountered many rejections because of their disability and lacked normal bonding. This makes them far more vulnerable to psychiatric illness in adult life.

Cognitive levels also relate to ability to cope with trauma. The highest level of cognitive functioning of a learning disabled person in Piagetian terms would be at the concrete operational level (characteristic of 7–11-year-olds) and many people with a learning disability will be at the pre-operational level (characteristic of children from about 2 to 7). This lack of the tool of abstract conceptual thought to aid understanding of trauma means that they are far more vulnerable to stress as they are less able to think through and resolve difficulties.

Are services available to people with a dual diagnosis? There is little data published as yet for the UK. However, Jacobsen and Akerman's (1989) study of psychology services in the United States found that information about client population was drawn from clinical history, observation and behavioural check lists, as well as clinical signs observed in making diagnostic judgements. Therapeutic interventions were aimed at a wide range of inter-personal and social adjustment problems. Any counselling was based strongly on a social learning perspective (Gardner 1967), and viewed as being most useful for people with a mild to moderate learning disability. Crisis intervention services were generally available, but not specialised services. Those with a dual diagnosis were found to have the worst service. Some 69–75 per cent of services were rated as poor or very poor, regarding either the existence or access to services which could cater for people with a dual diagnosis.

Allen (1989) points out that behavioural interventions which used to be limited to either developing self-help skills, such as dressing and toileting, or eliminating disruptive behaviour, are now frequently used to teach people with learning disabilities to cope with anxiety. The extent to which people with learning disabilities experience overwhelming anxiety, when compared with the average population, is very difficult to ascertain. It was mentioned at the beginning of this chapter that a lack of methodological consistency between studies has yielded conflicting data. There used to be a belief (Forrest 1979) that adults with learning disabilities rarely experienced anxiety to the same extent as people with average intelligence, but the move to community care may yield different data.

To summarise the main points covered so far, it can be seen that the incidence and prevalence of mental health problems in people with a learning disability is by no means clear. However, there is evidence that some people with a learning disability do have mental health problems and that for these individuals the range of services required are frequently unavailable or of a poorer quality than that provided to non-marginalised groups. Psychotherapy is one such service, and the next section outlines the range of therapeutic interventions that are available.

THERAPEUTIC APPROACHES

This section looks briefly at major categories of different kinds of therapeutic intervention. It is not intended to equip the reader with the necessary depth of knowledge and skills required to use these interventions effectively. Rather, it is intended to draw attention to their complex nature and some of the key issues concerning their use with learning disabled people.

Therapists have views about the nature of human beings. These views motivate their decisions about how to help an individual and affect their choice of a model of intervention from the variety of psychological approaches available (Burnard 1992). While many different models of therapy exist, they all have the common aims of improving the client's self-image and instilling the idea that he or she is a capable individual (Bloch 1982). This is in contrast to the commonly held belief of clients that they are the victims of their environment (Taylor 1993). Thus an aim of therapy is to encourage individuals to have an awareness of the impact they themselves can make on the environment. A further aim of therapy is to promote psychological and social functioning through the restoration and reinforcement of the individual's abilities to manage his or her own life. This also has the beneficial effect of increasing self-esteem and self-confidence (Taylor 1993). It is important, when utilising therapeutic techniques, to tailor the strategy to the individual's level of cognitive functioning (Williams and Mooney 1992).

The behavioural approach

This approach is based on the view that all human behaviour is learned, and as such it can be unlearned. The behavioural counsellor will identify what behaviours the client believes are unacceptable or undesirable, that is, behaviours which make the individual uncomfortable. Following this, a list of desired behaviours is drawn up and the person is encouraged to develop the desired behaviours. This approach does not attempt to understand the cause of the behaviour, and it can be viewed as mechanistic. The counsellor discusses the behaviour (not the reason for it), sets aims and objectives in relation to this behaviour, and devises a practical programme of small changes that will enable the individual to improve his or her coping skills (Burnard 1992).

Allen (1989) finds that despite the poor design of most studies, the evidence does point to behavioural therapy as being a useful technique for anxiety and phobias in particular.

In the laudable plea for far more respect and valuing of adults with a dual diagnosis, a backlash has developed against behaviourism, which is viewed by some as treating people like laboratory rats in an operant conditioning experiment. However, normalisation should aim at providing easy access for clients to all types of therapeutic approaches, including those based on learning theories, if it can be clearly demonstrated that behavioural treatments do fit in with this ethos.

Learning theories have been marginalised as yet another example of Western philosophy and science based upon the material and objective and are therefore often thought of as mechanistic and impersonal. Many therapists believe that learning theories view people as a mere product of instinct, heredity and environment and in response emphasise models which they see as increasing self-determination in people with learning disabilities.

Psychotherapeutic approaches

To approach problems from a psychotherapeutic rather than a behavioural viewpoint often implies a revulsion against the didactic approach supposedly espoused by behaviourists, and also that a relationship has been established in which the therapist is meeting with the client on the client's own terms. In this relationship the idea of the client 'being done to' is replaced by a 'talking cure' approach, in which authority is shared between therapist and client. However, the issues of power and control in such a relationship can be problematic. 'Meeting the client on the client's own terms' might imply the notion of participation, but underlying this is the issue of professional power. This needs to be addressed before the notion of participation can be promoted. Professionals, including therapists, concern themselves with social problems. As a consequence, they become involved in a problem-solving domain where the problems and their solutions are perceived as being technical in nature and therefore not political (Gloper 1975). This ensures that the problems and resulting solutions required belong to the individual. That is, it is individuals who need to change and not the social environment in which they find themselves. Taken to the extreme, this view can lead to a position in which individuals are seen as responsible for the manner in which society treats them.

Thus they are responsible for the rejection they receive because they have the label of learning disability (Menolascino and Stark 1984).

To return to the issue of the therapeutic relationship and the notion of participation, Arnstein (1969) identified eight levels of power relationships which are classified under the three main headings of citizen power, tokenism, and non-participation. It is under this last heading that Arnstein places therapy, implying that within the therapeutic relationship the power base rests very much with the therapist. This appears to contradict the shift away from 'being done to' to 'participating in'. Indeed the view could be taken that the behavioural approach is more honest, as the power base of the therapist is overt in nature, while in psychotherapy it is more covert.

Psychodynamic approach

The theories of Freud (Jacobs 1984) underpin this approach to therapy which focuses on the relationship between the unconscious and the conscious parts of the mind. The approach is termed psychodynamic because it is built on the belief that people are affected to a greater or lesser extent by unconscious motives or drives. People are unable to articulate why they are behaving or feeling as they do because the rationale for this is below the level of consciousness. This unconscious part of the mind is developed from past experiences. Some of these experiences may not have been dealt with adequately, in as much as they remain unresolved, and cause the individual to experience anxiety. When a similar experience is encountered again which can be related to the previously unresolved experience, people become anxious as they are reminded of the previous situation. Thus in order to understand a person's current behaviour it is necessary to explore that person's past.

Given the belief that unconscious factors affect the individual's behaviour, the therapist or counsellor will explore the client's history and help the client to relive painful past events, the aim being to reduce anxiety and thus improve rational decision-making (Burnard 1992). (For a discussion of the similarities and differences between psychotherapy and counselling see page 177.) The psycho-dynamic approach to therapy or counselling tends to concentrate on the relationship between current and past life events, and encourages the release of emotions which were not expressed at the time of the initial experience. The role of the therapist is that of interpreting behaviour, thoughts and feelings. However, the goals of psychotherapy are limited to what it is that clients want to achieve, and by what they are capable of achieving (Jacobs 1986) as it is thought that individuals may be selective in the recall of their past experiences. In addition to this problem of selectivity, people with a learning disability may experience difficulty with recall due to their restricted level of cognitive development.

Humanistic approach

This approach views individuals as being self-determining. That is, they are responsible for their own condition and are able to decide on their own course of action and determine what is good for them. They are not governed by the unconscious mind, nor are they a product of learning. The humanistic approach places emphasis on the individuality of the person and advocates a client-centred approach to therapy or counselling (Rogers 1986). The aim is to enable clients to work through their problems and to determine the strategies for doing this (Burnard 1992). The approach assumes that both the client and the therapist are trustworthy. However, a major criticism of the person-centred approach is that it does not address issues regarding the dark side of human nature and it is sometimes said to be naive and optimistic (Thorpe 1984).

Humanistic psychology, such as the Rogerian approach, suggests that the agent of change is the client. Clients are enabled to change bcause of the greater insight they gain during therapy or counselling. The aim is to help the client be more effective and self-aware through the personal relationship with the therapist or counsellor who must be formally accepting of the client, and show genuineness and empathy towards the client.

Cognitive approach

This approach maintains that the way individuals think about themselves affects how they feel about themselves. If people change how they think about themselves this will affect how they feel about themselves. It is believed that some people hold exaggerated and/or incorrect views of themselves and that this affects their self-image. These false beliefs can have a negative effect on a person's functioning. Thus self-concept is an important factor in therapy.

Self-concept is reliant upon the attitudes of others who are significant to the individual, and it develops over time. The need for positive regard from others is present from infancy (Thorpe 1984). Cognitive therapy or counselling aims to change they way people feel about themselves through challenging false beliefs. This approach could be seen as the opposite of the humanistic approach. The relationship here relies more on confrontation, uses a rational approach to problem-solving and encourages the client to develop a realistic practical outlook on life (Burnard 1992).

Eclectic approach

In the eclectic approach the therapist selects the most effective interventions from the diverse range available (Dryden 1984). The approaches outlined above offer different views of human nature. It is therefore believed that a single approach may not be suitable for every occasion, and that the therapist or counsellor needs to develop a range of approaches to be used according to the needs of the client (Burnard 1992). Goals are agreed between therapist and client which aim to assist the individual to develop psychological health. As with all forms of psychotherapy and counselling, a trusting relationship needs to be established. The therapist needs to be familiar with a range of therapeutic interventions and know the strengths and limitations of each (Murgatroyd and Apter 1984).

Some therapists use a variety of psychotherapeutic interventions even though they do not subscribe to the theoretical assumptions on which these interventions rely. They acknowledge the limitations of their own therapeutic school and enhance their psychotherapy by using techniques from other schools. For example, a therapist who is from the cognitive school may sometimes use techiques from humanistic therapy. Other therapists attempt to integrate two or more approaches both theoretically and practically; however, they may not achieve this. Combining approaches enables the therapist to use a wide range of interventions according to the needs of the individual. An example of this is when the behavioural approach is used in combination with a psychoanalytical approach. The behavioural approach will be used to change the individual's actual behaviour while the psychoanalytical approach will be used to ascertain and understand the reason for the behaviour (Dryden 1984).

Effectiveness of approaches

Psychotherapy and counselling as 'talking cures' are difficult to evaluate, as in practice a range of interventions are used. The tools used to assess how clients are before and afterwards also vary from study to study and some may be criticised on grounds of a lack of adequate norms against which results can be compared. Staff are often asked by therapists for their opinions on a client's progress as they may be able to express themselves more readily than clients. However, they may be entrenched in past experiences and consequently are unable to observe the changes which have occurred.

Skills for therapeutic interactions with clients

Accurate empathy, genuineness, and unconditional positive regard (Rogers 1959, Trauax and Mitchell 1971), have been identified by some psychotherapists as the most important skills for positive therapeutic interaction. These skills were assessed as far more effective than choice of therapeutic technique and may be present or absent in a range of therapists irrespective of the techniques they use. In other words, what counted was the manner in which they treated their clients, not whether they used behavioural, dynamic or any other therapies.

Empathy refers to how the personality of the therapist is an integral part of the therapeutic process. The ability of therapists to put themselves in the place of their client and to be able to see how clients experience their difficulties is extremely important. Empathy involves not just understanding clients, but also communicating this understanding to them and showing how much the therapist wants to help them.

Genuineness refers to the therapist being authentic and non-defensive in interactions with clients and unconditional positive regard means that the therapist is able to provide a safe and trusting atmosphere by wholly accepting and valuing the clients. These characteristics may make the ideal therapist appear superhuman, someone who never has that Monday morning feeling, never gets impatient or unsympathetic, and never ignores their clients' feelings. In reality, however, empathy, genuineness and positive regard refer to the desired characteristics of a good therapist, even if these may not be obtainable all the time.

This does suggest that people who cannot keep their clients' problems in proper perspective will not be successful in keeping their own personal problems from intruding into those of the clients, and as a consequence will be less than helpful as therapists. Indeed, such people may cause harm to clients by being manipulative.

Counselling or psychotherapy?

Some professionals offer clients counselling and others offer psychotherapy. It is difficult to differentiate between the two, as both involve helping people with personal problems and both involve being with the clients and talking with them often.

Counselling can describe a wide range of relationships, from the marriage guidance work conducted by Relate to counselling at a Job Centre in order to get a job. Whenever counselling is referred to in relation to psychotherapeutic activities, it has more to do with helping people with their personal adjustment. The term counselling is closer to normalisation, in that it suggests advice and guidance, whereas psychotherapy may suggest something far more intense, emphasising emotional states. There is such an open boundary between the two that there is little point in trying to separate the concepts. Although most counsellors may not view themselves as psychotherapists, what many of them do would be difficult to distinguish from psychotherapy. The main difference will be the scope or width of intervention.

Psychotherapy includes not just a counselling relationship, but also the use of a wide range of techniques to deal with specific difficulties, whether these techniques are behavioural, dynamic, cognitive or from any other school. Therefore psychotherapy can include the work of music therapists and art therapists, as well as the more traditional 'talking cures'.

Summary

It can be seen that a variety of psychotherapeutic intervention strategies exist and the choice of which strategy a therapist will utilise will depend upon his or her beliefs about the nature of human beings. However, regardless of the approach taken, the aims of the interventions will be to restore the individual to a level of psychological and social functioning which is acceptable to that individual. The issue of the nature of the therapist–client relationship is considered to be of the utmost importance. However, within this relationship a variety of tensions exist, such as the differing power bases of the parties concerned and the dilemmas that arise when the person presenting for therapy may not be the client. These issues will be explored in the final section of this chapter through the use of case studies.

CASE STUDIES

Angela

Angela had accused a bus driver of sexually assaulting her. She had informed her parents, who had contacted the police, and she had also informed the group home staff where she was living, and staff at the day service she attended. After careful investigation, the unanimous opinion of staff and the police was that Angela had fabricated the whole story. It was not this incident that had caused Angela's referral to the therapist, but it had coloured many of Angela's interactions with the staff, as she became labelled as someone who invented or exaggerated incidents in order to gain attention.

The referral to the therapist was triggered by Angela going out by herself to public houses and getting drunk. As Angela has Down's Syndrome, it was feared that her facial features would mark her out as vulnerable and that she could be abused by the men in the pubs who were buying her drinks. The sessions between Angela and the therapist commenced with Angela being very angry, spending most of the time talking about how everyone was horrible to her. However, she felt that staff had believed her about the incident with the bus driver, as she did not connect her perception of them as people trying to rule her life with their perception of her as someone who made up stories.

The therapist felt that what might be happening was that Angela had drawn attention to the bus driver incident as a way of seeing how people would react to her if she revealed sexual abuse. After a while, Angela felt able to describe a horrific incident involving rape which had happened to her a number of years before in a different environment. The rape had not been dealt with by the police and her parents had not been informed. Time was spent going over what had happened and how she felt about it, and the therapist moved on to discuss with Angela her wish to control her own life and her attempts to show that next time she would be able to fight off any would-be attackers.

Angela agreed that she was putting herself in an 'at risk' situation by her drinking habits and by going out alone at night, because she wanted to prove to herself that she could fight off anyone who wanted to attack her in the future. Thus an agenda was set for the therapist to work out with

Angela both safer ways of behaving currently, and also ways of helping her to come to terms with what had happened in the past. The therapist, owing to an agreement of confidentiality, could not discuss with other staff involved with Angela what she had said, but by attending reviews with Angela at Angela's request the therapist was able to promote the idea that by understanding Angela's reasons for doing the things she did that worried staff so much, the staff would be in a better position to help her.

Barbara

The second example relates to learning to understand the emotions expressed by clients during a therapy session, as these emotions can some-times appear inappropriate to those expected by the therapist.

Barbara was referrred following expressions of suicidal intent. The therapist expected to see someone in a state of distress, or at least depressed. However, Barbara came into the appointment smiling and apparently delighted to see the therapist. She denied any suicidal intentions and spent the session talking about a lot of different issues, including the fact that she wanted a baby. The therapist, who was heavily pregnant, felt that Barbara was saying she wanted to be like the therapist. As the therapist had to go on maternity leave, no interventions were planned regarding Barbara, although the therapist held discussions with staff who stated that Barbara often said dramatic things.

A year later the therapist enquired how Barbara was and was told that she was all right sometimes and depressed at others. The therapist agreed to see Barbara on a weekly basis. These meetings became very important for Barbara. Sometimes Barbara would arrive extremely angry with events which she perceived as being grossly unfair, and the therapist would listen to Barbara's story and gently try to aid her in problem-solving. The therapist was anxious not to offer Barbara a lot of advice, because she felt that Barbara's interactions with staff often involved Barbara being in receipt of well-intentioned advice. On other occasions Barbara would arrive crying and in an obviously distressed state, because of the things that had happened. Most of the time, however, Barbara would arrive smiling and pleased to see the therapist. It became clear that Barbara regarded the opportunity given to her to talk as being very important.

During the sessions the therapist began to realise that it would have been easy for people to label Barbara's presentation of herself as attention-seeking, or as shallowness of emotion, but that Barbara felt she could only get people to notice her if they were worried about her. Barbara was under-weight and was frequently sick and had many falls, which had resulted in scars. It was as though only by being ill could Barbara feel that other people would care for her. Therefore, together with other staff working with her at the day service, the therapist spent time with Barbara attempt-ing to increase her self-esteem. By aiming at showing genuine warmth and positive regard, the therapist used the sessions to show Barbara that she could be liked for herself, which the therapist hoped would release Barbara from the need to have other people worry about her.

Summary

These case studies provide examples of the complexities involved in the therapeutic relationship. The issue of who is the client is again raised, and therapists may find themselves in the unenviable position of trying to meet many people's needs which may be in conflict. Unlike in the general population, few people with a learning disability actually refer themselves for counselling. They are usually referred for this service by carers, which implies that the individual is doing something which the carers dislike and counselling is used to change this. This also raises the issue of the equal relationship which is supposed to exist between the therapist and the client. The question that must be asked is how can the relationship be equal when the person with a learning disability may not want to be there but will have been sent for therapy. This will cause problems for many counsellors, particularly those of the humanistic school.

KEY POINTS

Anxiety
Cognitive behavioural techniques
Dual diagnosis
Eclecticism

Empathy
Humanistic approach
Positive regard
Unconscious motives

ORGANISATIONS INVOLVED IN PSYCHOTHERAPY WITH INDIVIDUALS WITH A LEARNING DISABILITY

Developing Options Ltd
12 Church Street
Whitchurch
Hampshire

Fairfields Counselling Association
Cliddesden Road
Basingstoke
Hampshire

Tavistock Centre
120 Belsize Lane
London NW3

REFERENCES

Allen, E.A. (1989) 'Behavioural treatment of anxiety and related disorders in adults with mental handicaps: a review', *Mental Handicap Research* 2(1): 47–60.

Arnstein, S. (1969) 'A ladder of citizen participation', *Journal of American Institute of Planners* 11(2): 17–19.

Bloch, S. (1982) *An Introduction to the Psychotherapies*, Oxford: Oxford University Press.

Burnard, P. (1992) *Counselling Skills for Health Professionals*, London: Chapman and Hall.

Dryden, W. (1984) 'Issues in the eclectic practice of individual therapy', in W. Dryden (ed.) *Individual Therapy in Britain*, London: Harper and Row.

Forrest, A.D. (1979) 'Neurosis in the mentally handicapped', in F.E. James and R.P. Snaith (eds) *Psychiatric Illness and Mental Handicaps*, London: Gaskell Press.

Gardner, W.I. (1967) 'What should be the psychologist's role?' *Mental Retardation* 5(5): 29–31.

Gloper, J. (1975) *The Politics of the Social Services*, London: Prentice Hall.

Jacobs, M. (1984) 'Psychodynamic theory', in W. Dryden (ed.) *Individual Therapy in Britain*, London: Harper and Row.

Jacobsen, J.W. (1982) 'Problem behaviour and psychiatric impairment in a developmentally disabled population 1: Behavioural frequency', *Applied Research in Mental Retardation* 3: 121–39.

Jacobsen, J.W. and Akerman, L.J. (1989) 'Psychological services for persons with mental retardation and psychiatric impairments', *Mental Retardation* 27(1): 33–6.

Menolascino, F.J. and Stark, J.A. (1984) *Handbook of Mental Illness in the Mentally Retarded*, New York: Plenum.

Mulick, J.A. and Kedesdy, J.H. (1988) 'Self-injurious behaviour, its treatment and normalisation', *American Association for Mental Retardation* 26(4): 223–9.

Murgatroyd, S. and Apter, J. (1984) 'Eclectic psychotherapy: the Freudian approach', in W. Dryden (ed.) *Individual Therapy in Britain*, London: Harper and Row.

Reid, A.H. (1982) *The Psychiatry of Mental Handicap*, Oxford: Blackwell Scientific Publications.

Rogers, C.R. (1959) 'A theory of therapy, personality and interpersonal relationships as developed in the client-centred framework' in S. Kock (ed.) *Psychology – A Study of Science*, Vol. 13, New York: McGraw Hill.

Rogers, C.R. (1986) *Client-centred Therapy. Its Current Practice, Implications and Theory*, London: Constable.

Skene, R.A. (1991) 'Towards a measure of psychotherapy in mental handicap', *The British Journal of Mental Subnormality* 37(2): 101–10.

Szymanski, L. and Tanguay, B. (1986) *Emotional Disorders of Mentally Retarded Persons*, Baltimore, Maryland: University Park Press.

Taylor, T. (1993) 'Psychotherapeutic approaches with people with learning difficulties' in P. Brigden and M. Todd (eds) *Concepts in Community Care for People with a Learning Difficulty*, Basingstoke: Macmillan.

Thorpe, B. (1984) 'Humanistic approach' in W. Dryden (ed.) *Individual Therapy in Britain*, London: Harper and Row.

Trauax, G.B. and Mitchell, K.M. (1971) 'Research on certain therapists' interpersonal skills in relation to process and outcome' in A.E. Bergin and S.L. Garfield (eds) *Handbook of Psychotherapy and Behaviour Change*, New York: Wiley.

Williams, J. and Mooney, S. (1992) 'The wider application of cognitive therapy: the end of the beginning' in J. Scott, J. Williams and A. Beck (eds) *Cognitive Therapy in Clinical Practice*, London: Routledge.

Wolfensberger, W. (1972) *The Principle of Normalisation in Human Services*, Toronto: National Institute of Mental Retardation.

FURTHER READING

Brandon, D. (1989) *Mutual Respect*, London: Good Impressions.

Gardner, J. and O'Brien, J. (1990) *The Principle of Normalisation Programme Issues in Developmental Disabilities. A Guide to Effective Habilitation and Active Treatment*, Baltimore, Maryland: Paul H. Brooks.

Grunewald, K. (1983) *Emotional Responses of Mentally Handicapped People. Report of the Sixteenth Spring Conference on Mental Retardation*, Exeter: University of Exeter.

Humphreys, M., Hill, L. and Valentine, S. (1990) 'A psychotherapy group for young adults with mental handicaps. Problems encountered', *Mental Handicap* 18(3): 121–4.

Pedder, J. (1989) 'Courses in psychotherapy: Evolution and current trends', *British Journal of Psychotherapy* 6(2): 28–32.

Glossary

Beveridge Report 1942 This report was produced by a civil servant, William Beveridge. He was an influential figure who, working on the concerns of the time over national efficiency and political stability, produced a blueprint for a welfare state. The aim of this welfare state would be to remove what he described as the 'five evils' of want, disease, squalor, ignorance and idleness. It was Beveridge's blueprint which provides the basis for the development of the welfare state in the years after the Second World War.

Briggs Report 1972 This report gave evidence to parliament with regard to the nature and organisation of nurse training. It suggested a common initial training for all nurses, with specialisation towards registration coming in the later part of the course. This report, which saw nursing as related to illness, also proposed that mental handicap nurse training be excluded from its proposals. The Briggs report was never implemented.

Care management A concept previously referred to as 'case management'. This provides a central feature of the government's policy as set out in the NHS and Community Care Act of 1990. Care management provides a mechanism whereby an assessment of an individual's needs can be met through the purchasing of services from a range of service providers, the care service providers. The care manager, who is responsible for the development of the individual's package of care, should be independent from the providers of particular services purchased within the care package.

Charity Organisation Society This was founded in London in 1869 with the aim of overcoming the problems of providing relief within the Poor Law by co-ordinating the activities of the various charities. Previous to its inception a multitude of charities provided relief to the poor. This fuelled speculation about the existence of the clever pauper who would exploit the charity system rather than work. One of the COS's major contributions was the method of working known as 'case work'. This remains as the major principle upon which social work practice is organised today.

Consumer choice   This idea relates to users of welfare services having the opportunity to exercise choices over which particular service they wish to receive. It also relates to the users of a service exercising choices over the type and nature of service they receive. However, it does not necessarily imply that users will have any direct control over the way a service is provided, managed or evaluated.

Cullen Report 1990   This report, named after its chairperson Professor Chris Cullen, gave evidence in 1990 to the four chief nursing officers of the United Kingdom with regard to what it saw as the future of mental handicap nursing under the NHS and Community Care Act. One of its major recommendations was the idea of facility independence, which is the idea that mental handicap nurses in the future would not be based in residential homes. Instead they would work on a domiciliary or case load model.

Deserving poor   A concept first established under the Poor Law to differentiate between those people who deserved relief because their circumstances were not of their own making, and those people who had brought ill-fortune upon themselves. This latter group were referred to as 'the undeserving poor'.

Ely Hospital Enquiry 1969   This enquiry focused upon allegations of ill-treatment and other irregularities at a mental handicap hospital in Wales.

Eugenics   This movement was very influential in the mid-nineteenth century and the early part of the twentieth century. It was concerned with the control of human mating, with the aim of preserving or improving particular racial qualities it considered as beneficial to society. This movement also sought to remove qualities such as mental deficiency, which it saw as dangerous to the quality of the breeding stock.

Health of the Nation 1992   A government white paper setting out targets for the NHS in respect of improvements in health. This initiative sets out five key target areas for health services: coronary heart disease and strokes, cancers, mental illness, HIV/AIDS and sexual health, and accidents.

Humanistic psychology   A psychological perspective which is associated with the work of Abraham Maslow and Carl Rogers. The focus within this theory is how human beings make sense of their conscious experience. It is also seen as a reaction to the mechanistic approach to human nature of behavioural psychology.

Informal care   This refers to the care undertaken within families, and by friends and relatives, of people within their homes or within the community. Informal care is viewed as different from voluntary services. It often involves devoting long periods of demanding personal care to an individual. In this it is both emotionally and physically difficult. This type of care is predominantly undertaken by females.

Jay Report 1979   This report was produced as the result of an enquiry into the future of nurse qualification in the care of people with a mental handicap. It recommended that nurse training should be phased out with a new caring profession emerging that combined aspects of nurse training with those of residental social work. This report, which was a split report (a separate presentation was made by a group on the committee which included David Williams of COHSE), was never implemented.

Keynesianism   This economic theory, most closely associated with John Maynard Keynes (1883–1946), was very influential in the period following the Second World War. This theory proposed that the state could manage economic growth and unemployment through intervening in the economic system. It was upon this theory that the welfare state was developed. In proposing direct state intervention into the economic system, this theory can be seen as distinctly different from *laissez-faire*.

Kilbrandon Report 1964   This report, closely linked with the results of reforms in the care of juvenile delinquents in Scotland, reported upon the organisation of social services. Its recommendations led to the setting up of comprehensive social work departments by the local authorities. This was achieved through the Social Work (Scotland) Act 1968.

Laissez-faire   A political philosophy, associated with Adam Smith (1723–90), which insisted upon a rigorous and formal separation of the economic and political systems.

New Right   This political philosophy, most closely associated with the politics of Margaret Thatcher and the economics of Milton Friedman, became very influential in the period following the mid-1970s. It is characterised by a reduction in the role of the state as a provider, and a reliance upon the market to resolve issues of supply and demand. This includes health and social care.

NHS and Community Care Act 1990   This act arose out of a combination of concerns. The first concern was over the pace, organisation and funding of the policy towards community care and the closure of the large institutions. This led to a report by Sir Roy Griffiths in 1988 which suggested a greater role for local authorities, and the private and voluntary sectors. The second concern arose out of a crisis of funding in acute services which led to a series of embarrassments for the government. The result was the NHS Review of 1989 which set out the basis for NHS trusts, an internal market for health care, GP fundholding practices, and the purchaser–provider split.

Object–subject   This refers to a distinction made in philosophy between the subjective experience of human beings (subject) and the physical elements in the world (object). Subjective experience refers to the way in which meaning is created and experience interpreted through human interaction and reflection. To treat people as object is to relate to them as mere physical entities and to deny their essential human nature which is located within the subject.

Paternalism   This refers to the behaviour of a government or an organisation that can be seen to be authoritarian but at the same time benevolent. In health services this is seen in the way services or professionals respond when they act on behalf of a person. Here they provide a service to the person based on a professional definition of need. This would not involve the individual in either the definition of needs or in the evaluation of outcomes.

Patient's Charter   This initiative emerged from Prime Minister John Major's general initiative referred to as the Citizen's Charter. The Patient's Charter aimed to set out some basic standards in health care with respect to issues such as customer management, waiting lists, and response times. However, patients who find that their treatment does not comply to these standards do not have recourse to legal process.

Protestant work ethic   This idea, associated with the work of Max Weber (1864–1920), sets out the proposition that the demands of the capitalist economic system are closely intertwined with the religious philosophy of Protestantism. The work ethic sets up the values of work for the morality of both the individual and to society. In contrast idleness is seen as immoral, an idea associated with the idea of the undeserving poor.

Seebohm Report 1968   This reported upon the organisation of local authority and allied social services in England and Wales. The report was critical of the lack of co-ordination between different departments where social work services were based, i.e. child care, hospital social workers, housing departments. Its recommendations were for integrated social service departments to be set up under the local authority. This reorganisation, which brought together a diverse range of specialist social work functions, set up the possibility for the development of generic social work practice.

Special hospitals   These hospitals (Ashurst, Rampton, Carstairs, Broadmoor), which have been closely linked with the prison service, provide secure accommodation for a range of inpatients, some of who, but not all, have been convicted of criminal acts.

User participation   This refers to the involvement of service users in the ongoing provision of services. Here users are seen as having a primary role in the way services are provided, managed and evaluated. This model is often offered as an alternative to consumerist models of the provision of welfare services.

Welfare consumerism   This movement sought to make welfare services more responsive to the needs of users through the introduction of market ideas such as consumer choice, quality, information and complaints procedures. However, it is different from user participation in that the latter focuses on the involvement of users in the provision of a service.

Name index

Subject index

References to glossary definitions are indicated by **bold numbers**